Psychiatric

Examination

of Children

Psychiatric Examination of Children

JAMES E. SIMMONS, M.D.

Arthur B. Richter Professor and
Director of Child Psychiatry Services,
Indiana University School of Medicine

Fourth Edition

Lea & Febiger

Philadelphia

1987

Lea & Febiger
600 Washington Square
Philadelphia, PA   19106-4198
U.S.A.
(215) 922-1330

Library of Congress Cataloging-in-Publication Data

Simmons, James E., 1923–
  Psychiatric examination of children.

  Includes bibliographies and index.
  1. Child psychiatry. 2. Interviewing in psychiatry.
I. Title. [DNLM: 1. Child Psychiatry. 2. Interview,
Psychological—in infancy & childhood. WS 350 S592p]
RJ499.S56   1987   618.92′89075   86-20174
ISBN 0-8121-1061-7

First Edition, 1969

Second Edition, 1974
  Reprinted, 1977

Third Edition, 1981
  Reprinted, 1985

PRINTED IN THE UNITED STATES OF AMERICA

Print No.   4   3   2   1

DEDICATION

To Arthur B. Richter, M.D., cardiologist, scholar, teacher and friend, who for more than 30 years has worked in many ways to advance child psychiatry in the state of Indiana.

Preface

In 1980, when the manuscript for the third edition was ready for the publisher, I jokingly commented that I did not think of it as the "third edition," but as the "last edition." Reflecting on that now, I remember being more satisfied with edition 3 than with the two previous ones, but most surely I did not believe it was a definitive text on the child psychiatric examination. I did think the material had been updated so well that a fourth edition would be unnecessary for another 10 or 12 years, and then, if a fourth edition occurred at all, it would be written by someone else. The reality is that society and the practice of medicine are changing rapidly. The printed word becomes outdated and quickly diminishes in its usefulness.

This text was primarily written for child psychiatrist colleagues in teaching and learning positions throughout the world, and many have told me how helpful it is in preparing for practice and for certifying examinations. This fact alone makes constant updating mandatory.

Many other child-caring professions have found the book useful in comprehending child development and ways that social maturation can go awry. Primary care physicians, especially pediatricians, have become more and more interested in the emotional and mental well-being of their patients. In contrast to only a few decades ago, the contemporary primary care physician comprehends and uses the biopsychosocial medical model in practice. Although still lacking in some quarters, the concept of comprehensive care is gaining acceptance everywhere. Physicians are forming groups and affiliating with nonmedical professionals, not only for their own personal reasons, but in order to make comprehensive care a reality. This text contributes to total care by focusing on the long-neglected mental health of the child.

The post–World War II "baby boom" is over, but there are more children because of the large numbers of the population in their childbearing years. These new parents are vitally concerned with the early development and the quality of life of their children. They are demanding and receiving guidance and assistance in child rearing from many professionals. These attitudes may not be so evident among the poor or the uneducated, but they certainly have caught on among the blue-collar and white-collar middle-class families. These people may not eagerly seek care from a psychiatrist, but neither are they no longer adverse to the idea. From the physicians they select for their children they not only expect help in times of illness and crisis, but also they want comprehensive care at all times and continuity of care when chronic illness occurs. It is my hope that this book can indirectly promote what these parents want and their children deserve.

This fourth edition covers some new and exciting research on family dynamics and ways to assess family disequilibrium. The *DSM-III* has been widely used for 5 years now, and the text illustrates its demonstrated uses and limitations in clinical practice.

In this edition we have gone beyond diagnosis into treatment. We have given much more detail about the treatment of the children cited as case examples, and we have obtained as much follow-up as we could. This is not a controlled follow-up study, and the children were originally selected because they illustrated a particular diagnostic technic or problem. Hence, the clinical material is heavily weighted with serious psychiatric disabilities and challenging treatment dilemmas. Most of these children have reached adulthood. Some could not be located. Some are doing well and some are not.

The author remains concerned about clinicians' selecting treatments on the basis of their own theoretical biases rather than on the pathology found in the child and/or family. The clinician's theoretical biases cannot be eliminated completely, but they certainly should not be the primary factor in determining the type of treatment given. Chapter 10 lists the various treatment modalities available and illustrates the way a treatment plan can be designed uniquely for each child.

In the final two chapters, we review our relations with colleagues in pediatrics. Suggestions are offered the young child psychiatrist on ways to work effectively and avoid personal "burnout" in a pediatric setting. Many of the long-sought-after improvements in pediatrics/child psychiatry collaboration are recounted with pleasure, but remaining differences and some new conflicts are also discussed.

James E. Simmons, M.D.
Indianapolis, Indiana

Acknowledgments

I am indebted to many colleagues, residents, and students who have assisted in these efforts to refine diagnostic technics and communication skills. The ideas originated from the teachers who guided me through my own anxious years of clinical training.

Since the first edition in 1969, the comments, both critical and complimentary, from other training directors and residents-in-training throughout the world have been useful in helping me find ways to clarify this material as a teaching manual.

A generous endowment for a professorship in child psychiatry by Arthur B. Richter, M.D., in 1978 has made possible some needed technical assistance and given much impetus to this fourth edition.

I wish to thank Dr. Walter J. Daly, Dean of Indiana University School of Medicine, and Dr. Hugh C. Hendrie, Chairman of the Department of Psychiatry, for their continuous support and personal encouragement of this endeavor.

The contributions and comments of all of the child psychiatry faculty of Indiana University in reviewing and discussing early drafts are gratefully acknowledged. Those faculty who covered my clinical, administrative and teaching duties while I worked in the library and in my study deserve special thanks. This fourth edition could not have been written without such help from Drs. Susanne Blix, Judith Edwards, Jerry Fletcher, Matthew Galvin, Maleakal Mathew, Richard McNabb, Peter Mohlman, Shardha Sabesan, Takuya Sato, Kevin Stahl and Barbara Stilwell.

I am deeply indebted to Dr. Marian K. DeMyer for her *carte blanche* permission to use material from her didactic course in child development and from her continuously updated "Profile for Pre-school Children" (unpublished), now comprising items from 14 standardized preschool tests. Her critical review of early drafts of Chapter 6 were also most helpful.

I must share much of the credit for Chapter 11 on consultations and Chapter 12 on the interface between pediatrics and child psychiatry with Dr. Morris Green, Chairman of the Department of Pediatrics, Indiana University School of Medicine. For more than 30 years, Dr. Green and I have spent many hours together treating patients in the clinics and on the wards, teaching jointly in seminars, and discussing how we can learn to do it better. These chapters contain no direct quotations from Dr. Green for it is impossible to sort out his ideas from mine clearly or to recall the processes by which we resolved our differences. In this sense, Dr. Green can be considered a coauthor for these two chapters.

I wish to thank Ms. Marchelle Woods and my wife, Kathy, for their invaluable assistance with the preparation of the fourth edition manuscript. We are fortunate now to have an office personal computer with a word processor. Marchelle filled the computer disks and cheerfully inserted the many corrections and rewrites. She also took care of many administrative details and meetings, answered inquiries and worked on next semester's projects to keep the office running smoothly. Kathy was an expert at the tedious job of proofreading. She tactfully corrected my spelling and gave advice on questions regarding grammar and style.

Finally, the patience and expertise of Mr. Kenneth Bussy and the staff of Lea & Febiger in the final editing are most gratefully acknowledged.

J.E.S.

Contents

1

PREPARING THE CHILD AND INITIATING THE INTERVIEW

MUTUALITY OF ANXIETY

At the first clinical visit, there is often deep anxiety in the child, his parents, and the examiner. Children and parents naturally may feel anxiety at their first meeting with a psychiatrist. All of us as psychiatrists also felt apprehensive when we first began seeing children. No matter how sophisticated in adult psychiatry and medicine the examiner might be, knowing that even very young children can completely control the interchange is disconcerting, to say the least.

While trying to appear calm, the psychiatrist who is new to the child psychiatric clinic must cope with a number of questions running through his/her mind. Will the staff laugh if the child does not go readily with me? What will the supervisors say if the child will not talk to me or does not like me? What am I supposed to look for? What if the child is completely incomprehensible? How do you tell the difference between sick and well behavior? What is a normal 5- or 10-year-old like? How can a relationship be established if the child is too destructive? How can one be "accepting" of a child's symptoms without appearing either to condone or condemn the behavior? Will one who is sympathetic toward a child alienate the parents, and can one understand the parents' position without antagonizing the child? What special knowledge and talent allow the rest of the staff to appear so calm?

These and a multitude of other questions cross the mind of every child psychiatrist and pediatrician in the early part of professional training. To be forewarned is to be forearmed. It is hoped that the following suggestions about the family's anxiety will also allay some of the initial anxiety of the physician.

The child's and parents' anxiety on their first visit may be a reflection of underlying family problems. Nevertheless, much of the manifest anxiety initially seen should be understood and handled as fear of an unknown situation. Knowledge about procedure can attenuate these fears and make them less painful. Therefore, one should not fail to offer the parents simple instructions on ways to prepare themselves and their child for the first visit. The exact words used by the parent will depend upon the age of the child and the parent's estimate of the child's ability to comprehend.

Parents are asked *not* to tell the children that they are being taken to a school to see a teacher, to have tests, or to see a nice man who will play with them. If the child is failing in school, this is common knowledge, as is the parents' concern about it. Therefore, the child may be told, "We are going to see a doctor to talk about your trouble with schoolwork." If the presenting symptoms are nightmares, fears, or general unhappiness, the parents should have a similar frank discussion of the symptoms to prepare the child for going to the physician. In general, it is hoped that, through open discussion, the parents can avoid stimulating feelings of shame or excessive fears in the child.

A mother's questions about preparing her child may reveal her own feelings in a symbolic manner, but it is not necessary to confront her with an interpretation of her behavior. It seems best during the intake process to deal with the reality factors of the resistance in an educational manner, leaving the less conspicuous and presumably more neurotic resistances to a later time of diagnosis or therapy.

INITIAL ANXIETY AND RESISTANCE IN THE FAMILY

Since the first edition of this book more than 16 years ago, there seems to have been a dramatic change in many parents' willingness and ability to accept psychiatric services for their children. Many factors have contributed to this improved situation, such as more knowledge and acceptance regarding emotional problems and the work of the psychiatrist, largely through the media, parent education programs and word of mouth. We have lost some of our mystique but have gained better understanding with less fear and shame. In spite of such movies as *One Flew Over the Cuckoo's Nest,* there is now less stigma to admitting that one or one's child is a psychiatric patient. Indeed, we seem near the point where parents denying or covering up an emotional problem in their child are frowned upon by the community. No longer need parents fear being seen by friends and relatives at the child psychiatric clinic. In some segments of society, they are more likely to be criticized for not seeking help when the child is obviously troubled.

Thirty years ago, we had a special "preintake" or "prediagnostic" interview with a parent, usually the mother, to explore the "need for service," define the "problem(s)" and allay anxiety. Ten years ago, we were discussing these same issues over the telephone. In the last few years, we have usually been able to have the secretary make apointments by telephone in a matter-of-fact manner. Parents have fewer questions, less often cancel or fail to keep appointments, and express fewer fears that the very process of the examination will have an untoward effect on the child or the family. Self-referral by an adolescent who had never before seen a psychiatrist was rare 20 years ago. Now, it is relatively common. In fact, our own and many other public clinics will waive the initial visit fee, if necessary, for self-referred children. Naturally, every effort is made to involve the parents as quickly as possible, for reasons of economics as well as a sound medical practice. The changes in the laws regarding age of consent for treatment and the right of everyone, "even" minors, to treatment have supported our adoption of less cumbersome and less restrictive intake procedures.

The families who come to see us now seem more sophisticated and better informed. Even more important, professionals appear less judgmental toward parents and have more confidence in their ability to engage the family quickly in a truly therapeutic alliance. In my practice, the diagnostic process is greatly facilitated by having a family group discussion at the very first contact. The details of the family group intake will be described more fully later. We began using the family intake for some cases many years ago and now use it routinely in almost every case. The initial family group meeting permits us to inform all family members first-hand about our procedures and facilitates dealing directly with anxieties, anger, fear or other feelings that might take the form of resistance and impair the clinical process.

Although the preceding comments are true for the majority

of families being referred, there are exceptions. Fear and shame
of taking one's child to a psychiatrist may have largely disappeared, but ambivalence remains high. Many reasons and feelings lie behind this ambivalence, such as economics, time required, anger and frustration over the situation, lack of family
accord or ability to make decisions, hope that "it" (the problem)
will improve spontaneously, cultural, social and ethnic factors,
and many others. We try to arrange a visit of the family—at
least the mother, father and referred child—as quickly as possible, to explore these sociocultural barriers, which are unique
to each family. If they do not readily accept an appointment
from the secretary, we return their call and, occasionally, have
to explore ambivalences or resistances by telephone. When parents ask whether we think psychiatric help is really necessary,
we tell them we cannot have an opinion about that without
meeting the child and urge them to come for at least an initial
family visit. If they refuse an offered appointment, we urge them
to discuss it further with their spouse, the child, their primary
care physician, the teacher, or other appropriate persons and
call us back. After all, someone, somewhere, must have had
some reason for suggesting the referral in the first place. We
can hardly refute that person's conclusions without some observations of our own.

OVERCOMING INITIAL RESISTANCE

In years past, our experience seemed to be that families from
rural or politically conservative areas were particularly loathe
to acknowledge emotional problems in their children and quite
reluctant to seek psychiatric assistance. This appeared to hold
true, irrespective of the economic or educational level of the
parents. Without some objective study, we are unable to say
whether such a premise was actually true and, if so, whether
the situation reflected fear and prejudice against psychiatric
professionals among members of the rural population or a bias
of the psychiatrist regarding country people. For whatever reason, my experience had been that people from isolated com-
munities often were reluctant to seek psychiatric assistance for
their children, frequently procrastinating until the situation
reached critical proportions and its seriousness could no longer
be denied. Many families from all walks of life react this way
about their children. Currently, we find that such behavior no

longer seems particularly characteristic of or common to the rural population. The following case example is rather typical of our experience today:

> The Z. family lived on a rather large farm, approximately 40 miles from the city. The secretarial notes read as follows:
>
> April 30—Mrs. Z. telephoned, stating that Debby, age 5 years, is a "behavior problem." She has always been hard to handle but the last few months have been worse. She (mother) has "a hard time pleasing her." The family took the child to their family doctor, who feels she may be "hyperactive." He did not want to prescribe medication because she is so young. Mother wants to see a psychiatrist as soon as possible. I explained your schedule was full and that it might be 6 weeks before you could see Debby. She did not feel she could wait that long. I gave her Dr. S.'s and Dr. P.'s names, stating perhaps they could see Debby sooner.
>
> May 5—Mrs. Z. called back, stating that the other doctors' schedules are also full and they could not see her until June or July. She would like you to see Debby and requested we call as soon as an appointment can be made.
>
> June 10—I telephoned Mrs. Z. and offered an appointment for 4:00 p.m. on June 22 for mother, father and Deborah. Mrs. Z. stated that Debby has been somewhat better since school is out, but they will definitely keep the appointment.

There was no particular resistance in this situation. The case is presented here as a rather ideal referral situation, which appears to reflect a rather recent social change. The mother acknowledged the problem, even before the child entered first grade. She sought advice from her family physician, who examined the child and supported the mother in seeking further professional help. Even though the child improved with the end of the school term, the parents did not procrastinate.

Frequently, parental psychopathology, personality problems or marriage difficulties not only contribute to the development of symptoms in the child but also become serious barriers to effective evaluation or treatment of the child. These families sometimes can be characterized as "doctor-shoppers." They seek consultation from many professionals but, for a variety of reasons, seldom follow through. The prognosis for helping children of such families can be rather poor. However, for the sake of the child, every effort should be made at least to persuade them to come to the child psychiatrist or clinic for an evaluation.

> George M., age 9 years old, suffered from school underachievement. The family had been referred to a local agency, where they received some family counseling for a few weeks and then withdrew. George continued to fail, and, at the end of the school term, they were referred to a child

guidance clinic. He was evaluated and the primary problem was identified as an emotional one, with individual and family psychotherapy being recommended. The parents were not satisfied and did not follow the recommendations. George continued to do poorly in school, and, several months later, they took him to an internationally renowned medical center in the Midwest for a "complete pediatric evaluation." Part of this evaluation included a psychiatric assessment. There were multiple problems, both in the past and in the current family situation concerning social and health difficulties for several members. George appeared to be reacting adversely to these emotional situations but, in addition, did appear to have organic learning disabilities as evidenced by rather extensive testing. The medical center recommended both remedial education and psychotherapy near the child's home. A referral was made to me on April 20.

May 5—Mrs. M. called to ask whether we had received the referral information and to make an appointment. An appointment was made for May 15.

May 12—Mrs. M. called to cancel her appointment. She declined to discuss the matter and merely stated that they had changed their minds and did not feel that they needed to see anyone at this time. She would not say whether the child was doing better or whether they had chosen another therapist.

There was nothing further we could do except hope that someday George will get the help he needs. Sometimes, if the school and/or primary care physician repeats the original treatment recommendations often enough, the family will eventually follow through.

Most clinicians do not like to have families come under some coercive pressure. However, for the sake of the child, we must put forth extra effort to work with such families. The following is an example:

Harold Z. was 6 years old at the time of the referral by the school. He had had a normal birth and early development, but, shortly after becoming ambulatory, he was a problem child, sleeping poorly, not minding, having temper tantrums, and he was now getting into difficulty at school.

The parents had had a stormy marriage with frequent separations. They seemed not to be aware of Harold's difficulty and quickly rationalized that he didn't have any more trouble than other kids in the neighborhood.

At the time of the referral, the father had been in psychiatric treatment for approximately 9 months and the mother had joined him with his therapist in the previous month. The psychiatrist had suggested psychiatric referral for Harold several times, but there was procrastination.

Harold was reported to be doing poorly in school because of fighting and poor attention. Frequent conferences with the parents, initiated by the teacher and principal, had apparently resulted only in increasing animosity between the parents and the school.

The parents urgently sought psychiatric consultation when the school principal threatened to expel the child if this was not done.

In the initial interviews, much time had to be spent listening to the parents berate the school system, but they did agree to the evaluation and, eventually, entered into a treatment program for Harold. (For more details regarding Harold, see Chapter 2.)

In the following example, Angela's mother was also suffering a mental illness. This probably contributed to the child's illness, but, more importantly, the mother's own mental confusion seriously impaired her ability to cooperate with the medical system.

Angela, age 7 years, had many problems for a number of years, such as somnambulism, "excessive" masturbation, preoccupation with sex, temper tantrums, bedtime rituals, dawdling and poor school performance.

The mother consulted her local pediatrician, who made a referral to the psychological services of a nearby university. The mother worried that the child might have "dyslexia." Mrs. R. had had a very stormy childhood, especially in relation to her mother. In her late teens, she had a severe psychiatric illness and was hospitalized. This was a very stressful time for her, and, although her child's pediatrician was aware of her own adolescent illness, she refused to discuss the matter with him, constantly pointing out what a good mother she was and refusing to believe that her daughter had any mental problem. The university psychology services recommended psychotherapy for Angela. However, a short time later the mother called the pediatrician, stating that she believed the answer for Angela was for her to repeat first grade. The doctor disagreed with the mother, and she agreed to let the decision for pass or failure rest with the schoolteachers. However, she insisted the matter of "dyslexia" be explored further. The pediatrician made a referral to the Medical Center Pediatrics Department. The child was evaluated, and again it was felt she was suffering a significant emotional disturbance. The mother appeared to have a great deal of difficulty understanding this, stating that she was "sure her child did not have emotional problems."

Finally, when the pediatrician and the hospital Social Service Department insisted, the mother agreed to have her child see a psychiatrist to "rule out any emotional problems."

Angela and her parents were seen for psychiatric evaluation a short time after the pediatric consultation. Angela was, indeed, an acutely anxious and, at times, quite depressed little girl with many concerns about her own sexual identity and mental competence. The mother was seen as suffering from chronic schizophrenia, residual type. The father was an extremely passive man, who was constantly preoccupied with his own physical health, although, consciously, he desired to be a good parent also. This proved to be a rather difficult case, with appointments being cancelled and rescheduled frequently. However, with persistence, an evaluation was completed and a treatment plan instituted.

Stephen J.'s situation illustrates the way that an impending marital dissolution can defeat attempts to get clinical service for the child, especially when the referring physician is unaware of the parental problems.

Stephen J.—The following is excerpted from our office records:

April 12—Dr. H. telephoned regarding Stephen J., age 5 years. "The child is very hyperactive and certainly will not be able to attend school if something isn't done. Both parents teach school, are quite intelligent and want the child evaluated before school starts in the fall." The doctor was informed that we would arrange an appointment as soon as possible.

April 27—9:15 a.m.: Telephoned the home. No answer. 3:00 p.m.: Telephoned again. No answer.

April 28—9:00 a.m.: No answer. 11:30 a.m.: No answer. 4:30 p.m.: No answer.

April 29—Dr. H's office called regarding Stephen J., whom we had agreed to see. The mother told Dr. H. she has not heard from us and wondered about her appointment.

April 30—Letter from secretary to Mrs. J.:

Dear Mrs. J.:

We have been unable to reach you by phone in response to Dr. H's request for an appointment for your son, Stephen. Dr. Simmons explained to Dr. H. that he would not be able to see Stephen before mid-June or later, unless he had some cancellations. We understand you teach and assume this would be a better time for you, also. Please contact Dr. Simmons' office at the number above so that we can work out a convenient arrangement for you.

May 3—Mother telephoned. (By this date, the appointment we had intended to offer per the April 28 phone call had been filled by someone else.) Mother stated that when Stephen was less than a year old, he "never slept at night." Even now, when they put him to bed, he is awake for two hours, talking. When he started walking, he was at a "constant dead run," fell frequently, hitting his head in the same spot. (They have had this checked and the doctor says it is OK.) He has never slowed down. They have discipline problems with him—he doesn't understand "who the boss is."

Three years ago, Dr. S., pediatrician in M City, did an EEG; said Stephen was not hyperactive but has a "very wide focal range." A psychiatrist who saw him (name not given) said he was very intelligent and had vocabulary and speech ahead of his age.

Mother says they can't get him to sit still long enough to teach him anything. They don't want him to get off on the wrong foot at school and want him seen by a psychiatrist now.

When Stephen was born, Father was in Vietnam and then in Germany. Mother was staying with parents and relatives, so Stephen was surrounded by seven adults, the only grandchild, and had much attention. One person has suggested that he "never had a chance to be a baby." Father came home when Stephen was over a year old.

Mother works 8:00 a.m.—5:00 p.m. and goes to school two nights a week. Sitter cares for Stephen and her own two children. Sitter says she has no problems with Stephen.

Mother says when Stephen is with children of her friends, he frequently starts trouble—she thinks because he wants attention. He also interrupts her on the telephone for the same reason.

They will come any time you set the appointment. Mornings are better than afternoons. They would like to have their first appointment in mid-July.

July 6—Telephoned the Js. to offer an appointment for Stephen. Father answered the phone and said his wife is no longer working. However, she and the child are presently visiting maternal grandparents in Oklahoma. He will call us back to let us know whether they can keep their appointment.

July 10—Father telephoned to cancel the appointment. Mother is not returning from Oklahoma. She has filed for divorce.

Stephen J.'s case must be classified as a clinical failure. There is no value in blaming the parents, the referring doctor or one's self. However, hindsight usually has "20/20" visual acuity. It is important for both primary care physicians and child psychiatrists to study referral failures to see whether such defaults can be prevented in the future.

Perhaps the parents willfully withheld important information about their marital situation or the referring physician did not try hard enough to get the facts. However, in rereading our brief office notes, it is evident that the mother's behavior is contradictory, to say the least. She did not try to telephone the psychiatrist and was not available at home, yet complained to the child's doctor about not receiving an appointment. On May 3, she related some rather serious problems, yet calmly asked for an appointment six weeks hence.

Under excessive pressures for service, most of us are relieved if parents are willing to wait. However, if we had put the patient on "standby" to receive a cancellation time on short notice, the child might have been seen. The marriage probably would not have been saved, but perhaps the mother could have been referred for services near her parents' home.

Child psychiatric clinicians are sometimes criticized for insisting that the child patients be brought to them. However, if one's geographic area covers a radius of 200 to 300 miles, the idea of home visits or school visits is ludicrous except in very select instances. The preceding case illustrates that initial parental resistance may be lower than formerly, but it still exists. It is incumbent upon the physician constantly to streamline his own intake procedures and to try to facilitate the child's entry into the mental health system in every possible way.

INITIAL ANXIETY AND RESISTANCE OF THE DOCTOR

As mentioned earlier, the initial anxiety and ambivalence often so problematic at or before the first visit do not rest with the family alone, but are shared by the psychiatrist. After the family arrives at the office, physician anxiety may become manifest. This was illustrated earlier by the novice's fears about the child's being rebellious, not talking or being incomprehensible. The examiner may be worried about his own skill and competence, or something about a family or a presenting problem may be upsetting to him. Such initial examiner anxiety is readily understood by all clinicians, but the novice must consciously try not to compound the situation by expecting the impossible of himself. Many children do not talk on the first visit, and this is not an ominous sign for the future therapeutic relationship. The differentiation of sick and well behavior is not sharply defined, and the examiner will distort the whole diagnostic process if he is intent upon making sharp distinctions too early in the evaluation.

One former child psychiatry Fellow who was queried about his initial anxiety wrote,

> It took me quite some time to realize I had had a great deal of experience at interviewing persons, even children, before coming into psychiatry. . . .
> It was difficult to learn there are not always magical questions to be asked. . . .
> The biggest mistake I made in learning to interview was letting the discussion run itself while I searched around for just the perfect questions to ask. . . .
> I became aware of my need to fill empty time (silence) which was distracting me from what I could learn about the patient. I overcame that by timing the silences with a stopwatch. After learning that these silences that seemed endless were only 15–60 seconds long, it became much easier to tolerate them.

Another colleague wrote, "My very first child psychiatric case was a probable incest victim. . . .

My main problem in the interview was avoiding passing judgment and handling my shock."

Another colleague, a woman and former Fellow under my supervision, responded,

> My first child patient was a 7-year-old, "elective" mute child. She had been visually exposed to sadistic sexual behavior imposed on her mother by her father. When I went out to the waiting room to get her, her mother separated to be interviewed by another person. The child clung to her mother's coat and gloves ferociously. In an attempt to get her into the office, I picked up the coat and gloves and we both clung to them. After a bit of screaming on her part and bewilderment on my part, she walked over to the playhouse, picked up the dolls, and showed them vigorously involved with each other with a lot of genital contact. Then she looked at me with a sly kind of grin. . . .
> I have absolutely no memories of what I thought or did during the rest of that hour. The shock sent me scurrying to the clinical chart, to the other people who were working the case, and to the supervisor and books.
> I recall the whole experience centered around the questions: how do

you communicate with a child without words, and how do you deal with fear when you are frightened yourself? In retrospect, I now realize that I needed only curiosity to be my guide. She, the patient, was my teacher and, if I could tolerate it, she would let me know the traumas to which she had been exposed.

The examiner must make herself aware of her own feelings in the interview and try to understand them. To deny one's own humanness is a serious mistake. Any lost time or forgotten facts due to brief periods of introspection are completely compensated for by immediate improvement in our ability to listen and learn from the patient. Viewing the patient as one's teacher seems like a good suggestion. Naturally, for diagnosis and treatment planning, we must learn as much as possible about the patient. However, an accurate mental status assessment requires that, for the time being in the one-to-one situation, we concentrate on learning "from" the patient rather than "about" the patient.

DIRECT INSTRUCTION OF THE CHILD

Even if a preliminary interview with the parents, telephone advice, or a family conference has been used, most children come into their first private interview without understanding the purpose of the examination. The child may have been too anxious, antagonistic, or distrustful to believe or even hear the parents' explanation. On the other hand, the parents may have been so anxious about the visit that they could not even approach the subject and have just brought him in, saying nothing or having given him only half-truths and evasions. Therefore, some preparation of the child on the first visit by the psychiatrist is essential. This is done in the first family conference and repeated in the first individual interview. (For details of how the author instructs the child, see the section "The Psychiatrist's Initiative.") In her book, *Psycho-analytic Treatment of Children,* Anna Freud[2] reminds us that child patients are similar to committed adults. They are brought to therapy against their will. They usually deny a problem or see it as something outside them and beyond their control. This situation, as well as their fear and naivete, contribute to the difficulty in accurately assessing the mental state.

SEPARATING THE CHILD AND HIS PARENTS ON THE FIRST VISIT

In Tyler's report[3], the staff and the family engage in open discussion of the family's concerns and of the clinic's procedures. During this group meeting, the child is told that she will have some sessions alone with specific examiners.

The ease with which the child separates from the parents has some diagnostic value. Difficult separations may be due to a pathologic tie between parents and child or to the child's anxiety in response to new situations and new people. It should be noted, however, that difficulties in separating the child from the parents can also be inversely proportional to the experience and comfort of the examiner. If the examiner is afraid or expects that he will have trouble, he frequently does.

Since it is not possible to know immediately the significance of the clinging behavior, it is best not to make this separation forcefully. There is certainly no harm in permitting one parent to accompany you to the playroom, with the instruction that he or she may return to the waiting room as soon as the child is reassured. On rare occasions, for either the mother's or the child's comfort, or both, it is necessary for a parent to remain throughout the session. By action and by words, however, the examiner should indicate that on subsequent interviews he will try to make this separation. In a few cases, this separation has actually been part of the treatment for both mother and child. Usually, by the second visit, separation should not be a problem.

INTERROGATION VERSUS NONDIRECTION

Planned use of the physician's time is extremely important. It is necessary to be friendly, relaxed and unhurried. If one assumes the role of an authoritarian interrogator, such as may be seen in some law enforcement agencies, it may produce uncooperativeness, negativism, and relatively few data. On the other hand, the examiner cannot afford aimless, rambling, nondirective chitchat, which usually reveals little about the child.

Interview sessions should be limited to 30 to 60 minutes, to allow for the examiner's own schedule, as well as to avoid fatiguing the child. At our center, students are expected to see a child at least twice and, preferably, three or four times for a psychiatric examination, with an interval between visits. No matter how experienced the examiner is, an advantage of at least a second interview is that anxiety due solely to the newness of the situation will be less. More important is the fact that it takes time to know a person, and it is rarely possible to make a complete mental status evaluation in fewer than two or three interviews. In fact, the less disturbed the child is, the more time-consuming the mental status examination can be. The author is always concerned that a relatively asymptomatic child may be withholding information or "covering up." The same can be said for court-ordered examinations or circumstances involving pending litigation. In those situations one cannot promise complete confidentiality, and the child's trust must be obtained at experiential or feeling level rather than at the cognitive or intellectual level.

PHYSICAL EXAMINATIONS BY THE PSYCHIATRIST

The performing or requesting of a "routine" physical examination merely to "rule out" organic disease is useless, because ruling factors in or out is a never-ending responsibility. Nevertheless, before visiting the psychiatric clinic, all children should be seen by their family physician or pediatrician, because it is essential for every child to have a physician who is fully responsible for physical well-being and for the commonly accepted prophylactic measures against illness.

A physician's report outlining organic illnesses should be part of the child's psychiatric case record. Beyond that, medical judgment should determine the need for physical or neurologic consultations. From the history or during the course of observation, the psychiatrist may raise questions about specific aspects of the child's physical health. Appropriate questions are then resolved by the psychiatrist's own further investigations, with the aid of consultants. A consultant can always give an expert opinion on a specific question but is as impotent as anyone else in definitively ruling out organic factors.

In a medically isolated location, it may be necessary for the psychiatrist to serve as his own neurologic consultant and perform whatever procedures are necessary to answer questions raised about the child's physical status. Eckstein[1] takes the opposite position, feeling that physical examinations should never be performed by one who is or intends to become the child's psychotherapist. In my opinion, the child psychiatrist need not abdicate the responsibility inherent in his medical background. He must raise questions about possible organicity and work with his medical colleagues to find answers to these questions. This kind of responsibility begins when the patient enters the clinic or hospital and ends only when he is completely discharged. I see no contraindication to the initial physical examination's being performed by the psychiatrist. However, repeated examinations because of continuing or recurring physical symptoms should be avoided because of potential transference and countertransference problems. Usually, the child should be referred to his primary care physician for such additional examinations and any needed physical treatments.

VERBAL AND NONVERBAL (PLAY) ACTIVITIES

In our clinic, we prefer to use a combined office-playroom setting for interviews. This provides a greater flexibility and permits the child to accept either the conversational or play type of interview, or a combination of both. Its secondary advantage is that each person may keep his work space as neat or messy as he chooses, and the administration does not have to deal with the constant query "Who left the playroom in a shambles?"

The psychiatrist's activities are designed to make the child as naturally spontaneous and cooperative as possible. I usually try the conversational method of interview, even with very young children. Nondirective free play should not be relied upon exclusively. Lack of interview structure can make some children more anxious, because they think that the examiner is avoiding the real purpose of the visit. Other children may quickly learn to use play as a means of indefinitely avoiding talking to the physician.

In either fantasy play or direct discussion, the examiner should encourage the child to take the initiative. Do not be so passive as to create a new anxiety in the child, but, so far as possible, allow him to initiate and direct the play. A suitable balance between play activity and direct conversation comes with experience. The activity-passivity ratio varies considerably among equally competent psychiatrists and also varies according to the examiner's estimate of what approach will be productive with a given child.

Many novice examiners, without realizing it, enter a play-room with a child and immediately go to the doll house (if they are with a girl) or pick up the guns (if with a boy). By this action the examiner initiates play, and the child will then reflect the examiner's fantasies rather than produce his own. Adults seem to have an uncontrollable need to engage in some activity when they are with children. The obvious toys in the room are usually invitation enough, though you might add, "This is my room. You may use any of the things here." (If you use a combined office-playroom, you cannot have on display personal items that you will not permit the child to use.) The explicit question "What would you like to do?" is out of place. The psychiatric interview is not a den meeting or a summer camp where children must constantly be doing something to satisfy their leaders.

THE PSYCHIATRIST'S INITIATIVE

If the child does not take the initiative, it often helps to discuss quickly with him the reason for his clinic visit. This is the examiner's obligation and his opportunity to prepare the child for interviews. The child should be asked what he was told about coming and then questioned about his fantasies, thoughts and guesses about coming. If he can give any information, he is asked how the actual experience compares with what he was told or what he imagined about the event.

If he does not know or was not told, he may be asked to guess why others might come to the clinic. If the child responds with any statements at all, it is then possible to correct any erroneous ideas he may have and allay his anxiety. If he comes up with nothing, he may be told that the examiner is a doctor who helps people with their troubles or worries and problems. Children come to see him because of worries or problems about their friends, their family, their school, or themselves. If the child does not pick up these suggestions, he can be told that his parents were worried because he does not sleep well, because he is unhappy at home, or because things are not going well for him at school, whichever is true for him. With delinquent children who are highly suspicious, it is frequently useful to say that we understand they are in detention or have been in some trouble and would like to hear their side of the story.

If the patient cannot or will not use such openings to talk

about the presenting complaints or other topics, it is useless to push questions or conversation in the initial interview. Most importantly, the child should understand that you are not an object to be feared. You are definitely interested in him or her as a person, and you at least know of the existence of problems. Mentioning problems early may be useful for dispelling the suspense about what the examiner knows.

Often the entire first interview is spent trying to put the child at ease and clarifying the purpose of the visits. With some children, anxiety and confusion about the examination are not problems, and one can proceed to obtain as much of the data, outlined in the subsequent sections, as time permits. The psychiatrist should remember that the amount of data obtained will often be inversely proportional to the amount of pushing or authoritarianism used.

COPING WITH NEARLY INSURMOUNTABLE INITIAL RESISTANCE

The author sometimes breaches his own admonition against authoritarianism.

> An extreme example is the case of Allen T., age 15. Allen's parents made an urgent call, stating that Allen had become violently angry and refused to keep his second appointment with the doctor. He swore at his parents and had begun smashing furniture. They had fled from the house and were calling from the corner drugstore. Mr. T. wondered whether it would not be best for just him and his wife to come to the appointment without Allen. They were asked whether they believed that Allen was homicidal or would do physical harm to them. They were certain that he would not harm anyone, but when he got upset like this they just could not handle him. They were instructed to return home and insist that Allen come for his appointment. If they could not obtain his cooperation, they should call the Juvenile Aid Division of the Police Department. It would be necessary for them to file a complaint in order that the boy might be placed in the Juvenile Detention Home. Once this placement was effected, arrangements could be made with the authorities to complete our examination of Allen. In about 30 minutes the parents appeared at the office with an angry but compliant Allen. The police had not been called. It took several visits to complete the study, but it was eventually possible to establish a working relationship with Allen.

Such strong-arm tactics should be the exception and used only as a last resort. Coercion or other forms of force are not favored, but they may be necessary if the child may possibly do some irreparable harm to himself or others. Fortunately, since Allen was referred some 20 years ago, our clinical facilities have increased, and we would now instruct the parents to bring Allen to our emergency psychiatric ward. Once there, we would decide whether the evaluation could be completed on an outpatient basis. In spite of the improved training and skills of the local juvenile police, we prefer that friends or family members, rather than the police, assist the parents in bringing the patient. Allen's case is unusual and is presented to illustrate extreme action that is only *rarely* necessary in order to make a thorough examination. Allen was a very angry and uncooperative boy, and our threat to use police action to control his behavior did not endear us to him. On the other hand, he did not become violent or mute, but excused the examiner for his (the examiner's) behavior on the grounds that he did not understand what Allen had "to put up with" around the house. He spontaneously reassured us that he would not actually harm "them," even though he felt like it at times. He caustically suggested that we had forced him to come in order to be certain we collected our fee for the time. Even though he doubted our abilities and our intentions, the situation at home was so bad that he thought he would keep subsequent appointments to see what we could do. Hospitalization for treatment subsequently proved to be necessary, but by then, we had gained Allen's confidence and he was admitted voluntarily.

DIFFICULTY IN ELICITING SPONTANEITY

Marilyn, age 8½, was brought to the clinic because of the severe school phobia. She separated from her mother without difficulty but, in the playroom, sat with a "frozen" body posture. Tears were in her eyes, but she did not cry. Her pupils were dilated, her hands trembled, and her speech was a barely audible whisper. Attempts to discuss the scary feelings of her first visit did not produce any relief, nor did invitations to play with the toys. After 15 minutes she did accept an invitation to go down the hall for a Coke. She drank it slowly and looked at the pictures on the wall around the building. Her body posture relaxed, but she remained too tense to talk or play. On the way home she told her mother that she was "really scared, but the doctor bought me a Coke and it made me feel better."

Sometimes it is impossible to relieve a child's fear of the examination except through gradual lessening of the anxiety with each succeeding visit.

SELECTING CLUES FROM INITIAL PLAY ACTIVITY

Permitting the child to take the intiative in the interview produces valuable material. Often the child may begin by telling you in words or action some symbolic illustration of his presenting problems, his feeling about the examination, or both.

> John, age 7½, was referred for aggressive behavior at home and at school. He rushed to the playroom the instant he was invited. He quickly took the guns and shot wildly around the room with vivid sound effects and descriptive phrases such as, "I got 'em! He's dead! You dirty ___!" He tried to shoot the examiner but was easily persuaded to fire at the targets and the doll figures. As the intensity of his play subsided, he began to talk about his father and the fun they had fishing, boat riding and playing ball together last summer.

In this instance, it was not necessary for the psychiatrist to become active or take the initiative; indeed, such was probably contraindicated. John appeared acutely anxious and demonstrated that he handles anxiety by overactivity. He further showed that his behavior can be controlled by mild prohibitions when he acquiesced to the request to shoot inanimate targets rather than the examiner. He also evidenced inner control by gradually stopping the aggressive play. This contrasts with the behavior of some children, whose aggressive actions tend to snowball in intensity and cease only with strong external prohibitions.

The diagnostician needs to learn to identify the feelings revealed by play and the sources of those feelings. Violent shooting can be a direct expression of angry feelings and, possibly, a defense cover-up for strong fear. In John's case, it seemed highly probable that both fear and anger were stimulated by the examiner and the clinic visit. Had John been asked directly to describe his feelings about coming to the clinic, he might have confirmed this hypothesis.

The fact that John's violent play subsided so easily with a willingness and a desire to talk about his father made the examiner feel that factors outside the clinic experience were more related to John's behavior. Usually, the examiner would have some history that would provide additional clues to the meaning of the behavior. In this instance, the history was not available until after the initial interview. (Such a procedure should be followed occasionally to sharpen interviewing skills.)

John's spontaneous, glowing account of his positive relationship with his father made the examiner suspect some problem with the father. It is usually safe to pursue any topic introduced by the patient. Therefore, John was asked to tell more about his activities with his father. When asked about situations that caused disagreements and conflicts between him and his father, John revealed that his father had died 6 months ago. Without a strong emotional display, plans for the summer recreation that never took place were reviewed.

John was a highly active boy, whose aggressive feelings spilled out but were brought under control easily. John was still struggling with the mourning process. His desire to shoot his fantasied enemies. and the physician, followed by a glorification of the father relationship, was a graphic portrayal of ambivalence toward the lost father. Child psychiatrists frequently find that strongly emotional and significant topics determine the initial play activity in the first interview. Equally often, the child may avoid these same topics for several weeks in subsequent interviews.

> An 11-year-old delinquent boy opened the interview by bragging about how much he liked to have his immunization shots. He spontaneously told about a doctor friend back home who permitted him to go on house calls and sometimes give the shots. Sensing his fear, the examiner volunteered that he would not be given any shots. The patient responded by saying he had thought that the examiner would give him a blood test. The examiner explained that he wished to talk to the boy about the troubles he had been having. The patient responded that there were some things he would not care to discuss. He then launched into a long discussion of legal procedures followed by a detailed account of the inner workings of automobiles.

This boy was not a car thief. Rather, the entire first interview was concerned with his fear and distrust of the physician and, probably, all adults. He also revealed that he had developed some skill in the arts of evasion and prevarication as a means of handling threatening adults.

CONFIDENTIALITY AND LIMIT SETTING

Limit setting and confidentiality are issues that the examiner must keep in mind during the initial interview and in all subsequent interviews during both diagnosis and therapy. The limits that will be set or enforced and the degree to which the psychiatrist can be trusted are problematic to the relationship.

On the basis of experience, the child does not readily trust adults, especially strangers. If you are trustworthy, the child will come to trust you. With some children, however, this will not occur until treatment is completed. When a child stares at our note taking or looks for hidden microphones, we should try to induce him to discuss his concern for confidentiality. One cannot swear to absolute and eternal secrecy about the interviews, but one can promise the youngster that he will be informed when we plan to talk with the parents or others and will be told in advance what we will tell them. In recent years, I have been including the child, especially teenagers, in the treatment planning conference. Even so, the child is promised and receives a preview of what the parents will be told.

Limit setting is such a personal matter, charged with the professional's attitudes and feelings about aggression, that it cannot be dealt with adequately on the printed page. The effect of limits on the productivity of an interview is probably dependent upon both the conscious and unconscious intent of the examiner, the timing, and the intuitive grasp of the child's need for permissiveness or limits, as well as the past experience and nature of the child's illness. If you consistently have unproductive hours, you may be too restrictive. On the other hand, if the playroom is always a shambles and the patient is in an agitated state after your interviews, you may be either failing to set limits or unwittingly stimulating the child to act out. In either of these instances, some first-hand observations of your interviewing techniques by a colleague or supervisor would be much more helpful than a printed discourse on limit setting.

INITIATING INTERVIEWS WITH HOSPITALIZED CHILDREN

Introducing one's self to a child hospitalized on a general medical ward requires a different approach from that described for the initial outpatient visit. Hospitalization can be frightening in itself, and being taken to strange places in the hospital can provoke unnecessary anxiety if the child is unprepared. It helps if you visit the child first at the bedside and introduce yourself. Has the attending physician explained the purpose of the consultation? If not, an explanation and the reason for the referral should be given to the child in much the same way as instructions are given to the parents for preparing the child. The term *psychiatrist* is well known to many children, but it is best not to use this term until the child indicates some comprehension of the psychiatrist's function. One can make a comparison between his own role and that of the attending physician. "We are both doctors. However, Dr. Jones examines your sore throat, or your tummy, or your chest, and I'm a doctor who is particularly interested in children who have problems, worries, or troubles. I do not plan to undress you or listen to your heart, since that has already been done, but Dr. Jones would like me to talk with you about some of your problems."

Usually, the children's ward presents many stimuli about which one could talk for a few minutes. Some inquiry should be made about how long the child has been there and the way he feels about it. If there is sufficient privacy from the other children, problems may be briefly discussed. It is our practice then to inform the patient of our plan for a playroom or office interview. She is told the time and place of the interview and given some instruction about the location of the office in relation to her own ward.

SUMMARY

It is not possible to cite all potential variations of the initial interview. The majority of introductory sessions with patients go smoothly, and, fortunately, patients are usually charitable about our blunders. Nevertheless, the initial interview is troublesome to the patient and the novice examiner, and, in some instances, it may adversely affect all future attempts to work with the patient. Hence, the physician can well afford introspective evaluation of his initial interviews.

The initial interview for examination usually provokes anxiety in both the child and the parents. This experience also heightens the discomfort of the examiner when he first begins his study and practice of child psychiatry. Advance instruction of the parents for preparing themselves and the child, along with simple reassurance, will usually lessen much of the initial fear. It is also important sometime early in the interview for the psychiatrist to offer the child some explanation of clinical procedures and reassure him about his knowledge of the child's problems.

Occasionally, initial resistance and anxiety may be nearly insurmountable. It is important for the physician to recognize that the anxiety accompanying the first visit may unduly influence the child's behavior and that one must be cautious about drawing hasty conclusions from the initial interview. Although a firm stand, or even force, may occasionally be indicated with a particularly rebellious child, a patient, easygoing approach is usually more successful than authoritative questioning.

It is the author's conviction that physical examinations or consultations, when definitely indicated, are the responsibility of the examining physician and will not unduly interfere with the establishment of a relationship if thoughtfully and properly performed.

Eliciting spontaneity in the child can be difficult. There must be an opportunity for both verbal and nonverbal activities during the interview situation. The examiner must avoid being so passive that the child is unduly frightened or confused, but, at the same time, children should have free rein for fantasies with as little direction and suggestion as possible.

Some illustrations for selecting clues from the child's play activity are presented. Confidentiality should be assured by both words and deeds of the examiner. The matter of limit setting during the interview situation will vary greatly, depending upon the personality and tolerance level of the examiner. Yet, if the psychiatrist is too restrictive or if he fails to offer the child any behavioral guidelines, the child's productivity in the interview may be seriously distorted.

REFERENCES

1. Eckstein, R.: Notes on the teaching and learning of child psychotherapy within a child guidance setting. Bull. Reiss-Davis Clinic, *3*:68, 1966.
2. Freud, A.: *Psycho-analytic Treatment of Children.* London, Imago, 1946.
3. Tyler, E., Truumaa, A., and Henshaw, P.: Family group intake by a child guidance clinic team. Arch. Gen. Psychiat., *6*:214, 1962.

2

INTERVIEWING THE FAMILY GROUP ON THE FIRST VISIT

Experience has taught us the value and significance of meeting and formally interviewing the child and the parents together on the initial visit. For both diagnosis and treatment, it is important to get to know the family members individually as well as to understand as much as possible about the transactional systems of the family group. From the standpoint of the child and parents, a group meeting with open discussion of the problem(s) does much to allay anxiety and enhance rapport. My colleagues and I have used the family group intake[37] almost routinely for 25 years. We have found that it not only speeds up the diagnostic process but adds clinical data that cannot be obtained any other way.

Over the past 50 to 60 years, child psychiatric clinicians have learned that a thorough understanding of the cultural, interpersonal, psychologic and biologic determinants of the family functioning is an essential part of the diagnostic evaluation of the child. However, these data are supplementary and complementary and in no way should distract from the main focus of this book, namely, the face-to-face mental status examination of the child.

HISTORICAL PERSPECTIVES

Who is your patient: the child, one or both parents, the family, the school or the community? This is an important question because its answer should profoundly influence your comprehension of the child's symptoms and your treatment approach. Most well-trained clinicians recognize the impact of these multiple variables on the child's development. This eclectic attitude among professionals has not always prevailed, and even today in some clinical settings, less clinician time is given directly to the child than to any of the other factors listed. Clinicians comprehend the impact of the environment on the child's development much better than they understand the impact of the child upon his environment.

In an anthology, Ruhrah[29] quotes the publications of pediatric physicians from the time of Hippocrates (460 B.C.) to the mid-19th century. Frequent references are made to what we would now call emotional or mental problems in children. Even Hippocrates mentioned night terrors and insomnia in young children. Metlinger (16th century) wrote about "bad habits, anger, hot-headedness, sadness, fear, coldness, anxiety and ill-temper." These ancient authors provided relatively little speculation about etiology, and their treatments consisted largely of instructions or admonishment of parents about gentle persuasive corrective measures and more careful selection of nursemaids and teachers (Oribasius, A.D. 400). Metlinger quotes Aristotle: "The soul of a child is an unwritten tablet (tabula rasa) upon which nothing is written. One may, however, write upon it what one will." Kanner[18] notes that little serious thought was given to the causes of nervousness and mental aberration in children prior to 1900. With the advent of intelligence testing in the first decade of the 20th century, intellectual factors were given consideration as an etiologic agent in childhood disorders. The soaring interest in the childhood of adult mental patients confirmed what we apparently had "suspected" for centuries, namely, that the early parenting experiences are crucial to development. In America serious study of and work with childhood disorders began with the Witmer Child Mental Health Project in Philadelphia (1905), the Illinois Institute for Juvenile Research (1909) and the so-called Child Guidance Movement.[10] Juvenile courts began placing children outside the home as a logical form of treatment. Although parental counseling as a form of treatment had been used since Hippocrates and before, it was not until the 1920s that searching investigations of interpersonal relations at home and at school began to appear.[23] These studies were based largely on histories taken from mothers who brought the children to clinics, parent attitude surveys and some direct mother-child observations. Children were assessed professionally but not worked with directly in treatment until the 1940s. Fathers were not consistently included in case evaluations or research projects until the 1950s.

Kanner[18] states, "Even Freud, who so clearly understood the influence of early childhood experience on emotional development, had his theory of infantile sexuality worked out and published (in 1905), three years before he ever saw one single child professionally." Even without much direct talking with children, professionals did theorize and try to understand the real importance of the familial environment in both healthy and unhealthy personality development. Child psychiatry, itself a "child" of the 20th century, accepted that parental behavior and attitudes were extremely important for both diagnosis and treatment. Augenbraum[4] reminds us that Klein[19] in 1932 and Anna Freud[11] again in 1946 expressed pessimism about our ability to effect changes in parents, although both recognized the importance of such changes to treatment outcome. Two crucial questions remained then, as now: (1) specifically in each case, how do events and situations within the family produce symptoms? and (2) how can therapy lessen or remedy these psychonoxious influences?

In the 1940s, a few pioneers began studying and treating family group interactions by meeting family members together in addition to individual interviews.[1] Many of their early reports were studies of families who included a young adult suffering schizophrenia. For child mental health professionals who had struggled for years with parent counseling, child placement, and individual, conjoint, parallel and various forms of group therapy, the family therapy concepts and precepts had immediate appeal. Most clinicians saw the family group interview as adding new insights about live family interactions as well as another useful method of therapy.

A zealous trend toward family group therapy as the panacea for all childhood mental disorders has alarmed some clinicians. Many authors[8,17,22,33,39] emphasize that the family interview adds to our diagnostic understanding but should never replace the individual interviews. McDermott[22] reminds us that the "knowledge of the individual parts does not explain the whole," and, conversely, "knowledge of the whole does not guarantee understanding of all of the parts." In a G.A.P.[16] survey of multidisciplinary clinicians in 1970, 28 percent reported that they always see the whole family and never use individual interviews. Another 10 percent reported they see individuals only, without ever interviewing the whole family. We would hope to find even smaller percentages in each of those extreme positions today. Malone's 1979 survey of members of the American Academy of Child Psychiatry found that only 8 percent never use family interviews for diagnosis.[21] Howells[17] deplores the "fashionable vogue of plunging into therapy" before a systematic diagnostic assessment has been made of each family member as well as the group's interactions together. The history and the direct examination of the child remain the cornerstones of treatment planning. The addition of the family group interview as a diagnostic tool permits us to see directly the interactions that individual interviews only tell us about. These transactional subsystems can be one, usually not the only, cause of deviant behavior or even intrinsic psychopathology. In addition, we find that, whether or not intrafamily relations are directly causing problems, they can be factors that may aid or frustrate the treatment process.

McDermott's "Undeclared War" between proponents of family group and individual therapy[22] seems to have ended. The vast majority of clinicians currently involve family members one way or another in the child's treatment. It is now outmoded for therapists to isolate themselves and the therapy from direct or indirect contact with the child's family. We no longer see parents only as psychonoxious agents from which the child must be protected. Family members can also be victims of stressful interactional subsystems within their own households and can be seriously stressed by the child's emotional symptoms. Skilled therapists must lead parents toward becoming facilitators of healthy development of the child.

My own research[34] illustrates my belief that the involvement of fathers as well as mothers in the treatment is significantly related to treatment outcome. Even though this study has never been replicated, I feel distressed at how often clinicians, even those we have trained here at this Center, permit fathers to be excused or to eliminate themselves from the therapy. In my own practice fewer than 5 percent of fathers are not seen on some regular basis. This may be due in part to the fact that over the years my caseload has come to be made up mostly of professional and upper-middle-class families. I prefer to think that the involvement of my patients' fathers is due to my strong rejection of the archaic notion that child rearing is "woman's work." This belief is reflected in my behavior with and toward fathers. I have had one father who successfully evaded my insistence on attendance by going to sleep in the family group sessions. In 1968 Sager[30] reported on the problems of lack of understanding of the family treatment process as the cause of high absentee rate among lower-socioeconomic-status families. It is assumed but has not been objectively demonstrated that an initial, more vigorous educational effort with these families could lessen absenteeism. Teisman[36] reviews specific strategies for getting reluctant family members (usually the father) into the treatment. Among other points, he found that an indecisive stance by the therapist at the initial contact can contribute to the problem of involving all significant persons. In a 1978 study of "Factors Influencing Failures to Show for a Family Evaluation" Gaines[12] found no correlation between socioeconomic status and absentee rate.

DIFFERENTIATING FAMILY INTERVIEWING FROM FAMILY THERAPY

The beginner may be confused and feel that the differences between the diagnostic and the therapeutic family interview are unimportant. As is so often true of new clinical concepts and procedures, neither students nor teachers of family interviewing can yet evaluate its uses and effectiveness very objectively. In his most useful bibliography, Berlin[2] lists more than 100 selected references, mostly from 1960 to 1976, dealing with family interaction and family treatment.

There is no doubt that family group therapists have given us new insights into the specific relevance of family dynamics to deviant behavior. They have further shown another and sometimes more effective treatment for dysfunctional families. The novice may be deterred from family interviews by the erroneous fear of being immediately locked into full-scale family therapy. Conversely, the drama of the sessions and the frequently obtrusive pathology may entice the neophyte into attempting to change the family all at once. Both of these pitfalls can be avoided by carefully differentiating family interviewing from family therapy.[7,8]

The difference between interviewing and therapy lies in the conscious aims or goals of the interviewer (therapist). Every interview, ideally, has some inherent therapeutic value. However, the therapeutic family interview aims at changing the transactional subsystems of the family in specific ways for definite therapeutic reasons. The family interview, especially the initial one, aims at the clinician's learning more about the problems. One must understand the family's reality and the many factors that affect their readiness for help, the kinds of help they need and the form of assistance they can accept at any given time. The family interview is in some ways more flexible and open-ended than therapy. Questions and comments focus upon learning more, and the attitude of the interviewer acknowledges that the family is not yet committed to any particular form of therapy.

Grossman[13] describes an interesting method of observing families at lunch. The study reports that mealtime behavior is representative of family patterns of behavior in other situations. Although this assumption has some heuristic value, the subject sample is small and the data do not support the conclusion.

Selvin-Palazzoli[31] suggests three principles for stimulating families to produce meaningful information. He suggests that therapists use "hypothesizing," "circularity" and "maintaining neutrality." In a diagnostic interview neutrality is essential, as it is in family group therapy. Although "hypothesizing" (i.e., making unproven suppositions and checking them with the family) as well as "circularity" (i.e., conducting the investigation on the basis of data from the family) seem appropriate for helping families gain insight that will lead to change, these maneuvers are probably inappropriate in the early phases of diagnostic assessment.

Perlmutter[26] describes the assessment of families in psychiatric emergencies. Such situations can be very anxiety-provoking to the interviewer. In emergencies, diagnosis (assessment) and treatment (problem solving and disposition planning) must occur almost simultaneously. Engaging the family, reducing anxiety and identifying the request should be accomplished as quickly as possible. The focus should be upon the individual that the family identifies as the patient. The examiner needs a good grasp of social systems, i.e., the agencies involved or available to help. At the same time the interviewer must pay attention to the intrafamily subsystems, most particularly communication deviance. Emergencies often occur when the most experienced staff are not readily available. The interviewer must remain calm and allow himself enough time to avoid ill-advised actions or recommendations. One must have the flexibility to move from group meetings to individual interviews and back to the group. It may help if the history reveals, as it often does, that this family has been living in a state of "chronic emergency" for some time. Should this be true, pressure for immediate action may be a need of the clinician and not a specific demand of any member of the family. One rather frequent emergency is child abuse. There are many things that we, along with our medical colleagues, can do for these children and their families. Yet it is rather common knowledge that resistance to psychiatric treatment and drop-out rates are extremely high.[28] In a 1985 study comparing abusive and non-abusive families with conduct-disordered children, Webster-Stratten[41] found no single variable that significantly discriminates the two types of families; however, low income, family history of abuse and maternal depression were more frequent in the abusing families.

Viaro,[39] using theories of conversational analysis, differentiates "treatment" conversation from "everyday" conversation. "Five Rules of Direction" distinguish the treatment interview. Viaro describes the rules as the "rights" of the therapist. We would say these are the obligation and duty of the interviewer as he controls and directs the conversation. However, the interviewer does not do more than ask questions, sum up and organize what has been said. Viaro does not state the rules to the family since they are "implicit" by his behavior. For me, the fact that I control and direct is also implicit by my behavior, but I prefer to state the other rules up front early. These are simply (1) Everyone can speak; (2) family members are asked to listen or hear each other out; and (3) interrupting or retaliating against those with differing views is discouraged. By my behavior I reinforce these rules. Viaro warns that the interviewer can prevent the flow of useful information by exerting too much or too little authority. It is not so much the behavior of the interviewer as his/her aims and goals along with sensitivity to what encourages the family to give information that result in a productive or nonproductive session.

Roberts,[27] Walker,[40] Olson,[25] and Beavers[6] all describe methods of assessing, describing, rating and classifying family behavior and functioning. Patterns of cohesion and adaptability are of considerable interest to investigators at this time. The methodologies are rather time-consuming and cumbersome for daily use by clinicians, but such research is vital to improving our understanding of family interaction patterns. Beavers rates both cohesion and adaptability along a continuum and proposes

nine family types from "optimal" to "severely disturbed cen-
tripetal and/or centrifugal" families. The family type may bear
a significant relationship to the psychopathology of individual
family members and have explicit implications for family treatment. Future research of these issues of family structure and
functions will be increasingly valuable to clinicians.

THE FAMILY INTERVIEW PROCESS

In the American Academy of Child Psychiatry Survey previously cited,[21] 92 percent of the responders said they used
family interviews in diagnosis. Even so, our literature over-
whelmingly focuses on family therapy. We did find a few ar-
ticles aimed primarily at the diagnostic use of the family group
interview.[9,20,32,33,38,42,43] Apparently, most clinicians have developed a unique approach by extrapolating ideas from individual interviewing to family group by trial and error. My technique for interviewing families closely resembles that reported
by Tyler[37] and Serrano,[32] although the latter seems to take more
time and have a less rigid structure. Serrano invites everyone
in the household; I ask only mother, father and child to the
initial visit. In the following example the reader will see that I
notice family dysfunctioning areas but my primary focus is on
the child patient, clarifying the reasons for bringing the child
for evaluation and teaching the family about the evaluation
process itself.

Some family interviews are quite difficult to arrange, and,
occasionally, it is impossible to hold such a meeting. However,
I cannot recall a single instance in the past 25 years when
something so unfortunate happened as to make the initial group
meeting seem ill-advised. The initial meeting seems actually to
protect rather than violate confidentiality. Furthermore, the
group interview usually lessens the child's distrust and resistance while enhancing the parents' confidence. The interview
can usually focus on the family's mutual desire to find real
solutions rather than just someone to blame. Family group meetings can be held at any point during diagnosis or therapy. We
prefer to have a family session on the first visit, irrespective of
whether or not such sessions may be used in therapy later. When
family interviews are introduced early, their intercurrent use
later in therapy is relatively easy and uncomplicated.

Most authors seem to agree on several issues: in the diagnostic session, encourage open discussion but do not force it; be alert and provide support when an individual, usually the index child, is put on the "hot seat"; be certain each person present has a chance to express himself or herself to the extent he/she wishes or is able. The following procedure evolved out of my personality and expediency of my particular situation.

Prior to the first interview, there may be much information available about the child and family from a referring physician, school or other agency. Most often, however, the only information we have are the presenting complaint and a few demographic items that the secretary recorded when the parent called for an appointment. The following is an example of an initial family group interview.

CASE EXAMPLE*

Request for Appointment

(Information taken by secretary per phone) Date: 11/17/79

Patient:	Harold Z., Jr.	D.O.B. 12/19/72	Age 6 years, 11 months
Parents:	Harold, Sr.	Marybeth	
	Father	Mother	

Address: Parents live together at a rural address near a small town (population under 3,000)

Referred by: Dr. M.S.K. (psychiatrist)

Problem: He is a behavior problem in school (first grade); noisy, doesn't get along with classmates. Teacher says he will have to be put out of class if he doesn't change. Hyperactive?

He was given some sort of test at school (the mother couldn't remember what it was), and results indicated he should be seen by a psychiatrist "as soon as possible."

Dr. S.'s notes to secretary: Have parents instruct school to send report of their evaluation. Schedule both parents and child as soon as there's an opening in my calendar.

School Report

(Arrived prior to first appointment)

Mayfair School	John Smith, Principal
Harold Z.	6 yrs. 9 mos., in first grade

Tested by Ellen Jones, certified psychometrist 9/79

Test	*Results*	
WISC-R	Verbal IQ	89
	Performance IQ	89
	Full-Scale IQ	89

---

*The office procedures and interview techniques are my own. For purposes of conciseness and clarity, my own and others' variations are not recounted. The reader should consult the literature and his own intuitive senses to find procedures and technics that are productive yet more suitable to his personality and clinical environment. One should not blindly follow my examples.

Wide Range Achievement Test	Grade Level
Spelling	Kindergarten: 9th month
Math	Kindergarten: 9th month
Reading	Kindergarten: 8th month

Beery Developmental Test of Visual Motor Integration

Functioning equivalent to average 5-year, 3-month child

Bender-Gestalt

Within normal limits developmentally

Draw a Human Figure

Figure very small: less than 1 inch on an 8½ × 11 sheet of paper
No body
No arms

Conclusion: The testing results indicate Harold may be a slow learner. Family counseling was recommended as the school feels the situation at home might be at the root of the problem. The older brother (age 12) was a big behavior problem in grade school. The principal said he was "the worst kid he had ever had." The sister (age 10) is having some social problems with her peers.

Harold's teacher says he has to be forced to do any work at all. He has trouble with his peers, fights, and spits. He reverses his writing and numbers. Testing shows hearing loss. It was recommended that the teacher give as much positive feedback as possible to Harold, praise him, and encourage him to join in activities.

First Psychiatric Visit

Initial Interview

(In the interest of space and because it was not tape-recorded, much of the dialogue has been condensed and paraphrased.)

Mother, father, and child arrived on time. All were sitting in the waiting room, stone-faced, leafing through magazines.

Dr. S. introduced himself, shook hands all around and, looking at Harold, said: "I'd like to start with all of us together in my office to talk about why you came to see me. After that, Harold, you and I can visit alone for a while."

Family was taken to the office. Usually, the author begins by talking to the child to try to put him at his ease and to find out how he was prepared for the initial visit. However, in this instance, the mother was very tense and began talking even before everyone was seated.

MO.: He's been misbehaving in school. Here! (holds out a sheaf of note papers). I get four or five of these every week. He gets whacks from the principal every day.

DR. S.: (Glances briefly at the school notes, which seemed to list the offenses of the day.) May I keep these to look over more closely before your next appointment? (Looks at child who's sitting on edge of chair.) Harold, we'll have an appointment every week for the next few weeks. Sometimes we'll all talk together, but, usually, I'll see each of you alone. I need to get to know you, Mom and Dad and learn about the troubles you've been having. When I feel I understand things, we'll meet again and talk about what can be done to make things better.

HAROLD: (Stares at the floor and holds the arms of the chair tightly.)

DR S.: You look kind of scared. Was it scary coming here today?

MO. (interrupts): The school said he's dull normal. I want his tests repeated. I think he's much better than that.

DR. S. (to Harold): Have things been pretty unhappy for you at school?

MO. (interrupts): It all started 3 weeks ago. Mr. S. (principal) called for a conference. He said Harold would have to go to special classes for disturbed children or they'd expel him. Then 2 weeks ago the school counselor said they disagreed. A lot of parents are dissatisfied with that school. The teachers don't get along with each other. Seems they don't know what they're doing. They tell you a lot of different things or don't tell you anything. Then they say they're gonna expel him. I just don't know. (deep breath).

He's OK at home (meaning Harold). Maybe a little overactive. The only problem is getting him to school. He balks and won't go unless I take him. I have to take him about every day. He won't even dress himself. I have to dress him and take him to school. That principal is an awful person. No one likes him, not even the teachers. He doesn't understand children. He told me I didn't handle Harold right (deep breath).

DR. S. (catching Harold's intent expression): Harold, did you want to say something?

HAROLD: Mr. S. whacks me. Jerry pushed me down on the playground.

MO. (interrupts): The school denies that ever happened.

DR. S. (to Harold): Do you want to tell me about it?

HAROLD: I didn't do nothing but I got whacked.

DR. S.: How'd you feel?

HAROLD: I didn't like getting whacked.

DR. S.: Then what happened?

HAROLD: I had to go sit on the bench and then go to class.

DR. S.: What were you feeling then?

MO. (breaks silence): Mr. Z. has been in treatment with Dr. M.S.K. (psychiatrist) for the past 9 months. I started seeing him, too, a month ago.

DR. S.: (waits expectantly; silence).

MO.: He's been no problem around home (meaning Harold). (Mother continues berating the school system with many examples that had been furnished by her friends; silence.)

FA.: We had problems with his older brother, Billy. Billy had a learning problem and was operated on by Dr. W. (otolaryngologist). Mr. S., the principal, accused Billy of being a behavior problem, too. (Mr. Z then launches into a lengthy monologue expressing dissatisfaction with the town where they live. The schools are inadequate, as are the other government services and officials. Everybody in the town is dissatisfied, even the kids. They can't seem to get along. They fight all the time. Occasionally, he mentions Harold's temper tantrums, failure to obey, and fighting. However, he concludes that the entire town fights all the time and Harold is no worse than any of the others.)

Mr. Z seems rather depressed but cannot or will not identify any problem except those outside his family. Perhaps he is just ventilating feelings. From the content of his talk, he appears to acknowledge Harold's problems. However, he resents what he perceives as the school's attitude toward his family. He projects his feelings of anger and distrust onto the community. Mother, father and child seem to be struggling with intense anger, which they aim at people outside the home. They do not display anger toward each other. They admit Harold's problems but resist any

full description by minimizing and denying. Fear of revealing
the marital situation may have contributed much to this resistance. It seems to the examiner that any interpretation or too much
pressure for details would run the risk of increasing the resistance
or even alienating them. They also interrupt each other and
change the subject so frequently that it is hard to follow what
they are saying. It seems unlikely that a coherent description of
Harold's problems will be forthcoming. Therefore, a more structured, straight history-taking approach is tried.

DR. S. (looking at his watch): We're running out of time. Before I see Harold
alone, there are several questions I need to ask about his development that he can't answer. Tell me about the pregnancy and
delivery with him. (From straight fact-gathering questions it is
learned that the parents have been married 14 years and have a
boy age 12 and a girl age 10 years. There have been no miscar-
riages and no previous marriages. Harold's pregnancy was
planned and full-term without complications. Delivery was normal. Birth weight was 6 pounds, 8 ounces. The neonatal period
went well. He cried very little and was an "independent" baby.
Developmental milestones were poorly recalled but mother remembered, "He walked at 7 months, swam in the creek at age 2
years and was talking well before 2 years of age." Mother's health
during pregnancy was good. Postpartum depression is denied.
They are asked about problems with grandparents, personal
health, nervousness or depression in themselves. In response to
the last question, mother replies, "Harold is lazy. We do too much
for him. He won't dress himself; he waits 'til I do it for him. He
does have temper tantrums. He kicks the wall and yells."

Attempts to get a better description of the tantrums and how
they were handled produce rather vague, evasive answers. It is
assumed she is still not ready to talk about Harold's problems
but is merely trying to avoid my earlier personal questions about
her and her husband.

They are asked to tell about their current treatment with the
referring psychiatrist. They decline. Although Harold knows they
are getting psychiatric help, it does not involve him. They are
asked whether there had ever been separations due to military
service, job changes or personal problems. Mother says she has
left several times with the children, but reconciliation has always
occurred. The separations have lasted from three weeks to two
months. The last separation occurred six months ago.

*(Note: The author prefers the open-ended, exploratory-type
interview because it usually can produce more information about
subtle and spontaneous family interactions, more easily reveals
the uniqueness of each family and permits a preliminary assessment of the family's readiness for treatment. This family is
so tense and resistive that we switched to the more structured
history-taking type questions. We hope this will lessen anxiety,
reveal a few facts and also serve to educate them regarding areas
that the examiner considers important.)*

DR. S.: Well, our family session has gone longer than I intended. We
can go into more details of these many important issues at future
appointments but, just now, I need to see Harold alone for the
remainder of the time.

*(Note: Some time alone with Harold appears to be important.
The parents seem able to accept him as the primary patient, and*

I do not wish to leave the impression that family pathology is my sole interest. More importantly, Harold has remained very tense and nearly unable to talk. I hope I can help him relax before leaving. The parents leave for the waiting room.)

DR. S. (pointing to the open doors of the cupboard and closet): There are lots of my things in there. You can use them if you like. (Harold begins exploring.)

DR. S.: Did it upset you some to have to sit there while Mom and Dad talked about all these things?

HAROLD (retrieving a dart game from the cupboard): I learned all my numbers in school: 1, 2, 3, 4, 5, 6, etc., etc. (He stops at 20, having made two mistakes that he does not recognize. Harold hands the examiner two blue darts and keeps the two red ones for himself. It is decided that a score of 100 will be game. Harold is not fearful and is quite accurate with the darts.)

DR. S.: Do you have some private worries you didn't want to tell in front of your parents?

HAROLD: Dad comes home drunk a lot. They fight.

DR. S.: Is that scary?

HAROLD: They just yell a lot. Sometimes he leaves.

DR. S.: You want to tell me about it? (With minimal encouragement, Harold reveals that mother takes him and his siblings to his aunt's house. He doesn't like it there. Her kids are mean and they fight him. He worries that something bad will happen to his dad. They've been fighting about every day lately, and he's scared mother is going to leave. He's too afraid to tell them how he feels. He gets mad, too, but he doesn't show it. He just goes out to play and forgets it.

Two more dart games are played and then Harold is told the time is up and that he will talk more about his worries next time.)

Initial Impressions

From the school report and this interview, Harold may have a school learning problem that is complicated by a serious marital disorder and, possibly, paternal alcoholism. So far, there are no obvious signs of serious physical disorder or psychosis in any of the three persons interviewed.

Diagnostic Plan

1. Get pediatrician's report, including examination of hearing and vision.
2. Neurologic consultation probably not needed. Will do a neurologic screening myself.
3. Complete the mental status examination of Harold. Will try to determine whether behavior problems are "reactive" or whether deeper character pathology is present.
4. Get a description of the marital situation from each parent.
5. Personal history and mental status assessment of each parent. May get Minnesota Multiphasic Personality Inventory (MMPI) later on each parent.
6. Get report from the parents' psychiatrist.

Author's Note:

The reader will be interested in knowing that, in subsequent interviews, the "mean" principal and his "incompetent" staff are not mentioned again. The full diagnostic assessment was completed according to the outline given in subsequent chapters.

Summary

Harold Z. and his parents were evaluated over several weeks' time. Harold's achievement level was 2 to 3 months below his grade placement. His IQ was low average. History and psychiatric exam revealed that he suffered a conduct disorder, socialized, aggressive. Mother, age 32, was very unhappy, feeling trapped in a "hopeless" marriage. Father, age 33, had been placed on Antabuse for alcoholism and a tricyclic antidepressant. He refused to go to Alcoholics Anonymous and would stop his Antabuse when he drank. A socially dysfunctional 12-year-old brother and a 10-year-old sister were invited to join us for a series of family "meetings" to explore some possible ways of helping the family. The situation seemed hopeless, with constant fussiness, bickering and confusion. After two such meetings the mother left home and filed for divorce. The father took the children and moved to his parents' home in Florida. Attempts over the years to trace this family have been to no avail.

As illustrated here, both parents are requested to come for the first interview. However, a child is never refused an appointment if this is really not possible. Every effort is made to coordinate the psychiatrist's and the working parents' schedules. The hours from the close of school until dinnertime are frequently requested so "the child won't have to miss school." It is explained that this "prime time" is filled by children in therapy who have to come frequently over a long period of time and, usually, an earlier hour is necessary for the diagnostic interviews. If one parent's schedule requires him or her to be out of town during the work week, their actual work commitments are explored in detail. When the real importance of both parents' attending is properly conveyed, a mutually agreeable time can almost always be found. Stepparents and nonmarried mates living in the home with the child are always included. In divorced families, the noncustodial parent(s) occasionally may be invited to the initial visit if communication among the adults has been reasonably good. The need to include noncustodial parents at some point in the evaluation is always stated. Most often, the parent(s) with whom the child does not live are seen at another time. The child may be included in this second family interview if the contacts with them are frequent and regular, and the noncustodial parents are truly involved with him. The index patient is usually not included in the interview with the alternate family when there are hotly contested custody problems. Sometimes an appointment can be arranged during the child's regular visitation with the noncustodial parent. Although it is desirable to see the child interacting with all of his important adults, good judgment must prevail. He should not be unnecessarily exposed to loud emotional out-bursts such as sometimes occur in court custody or divorce hearings.

If possible, foster parents* are interviewed on the first visit with the child. In such cases, the biological parents are seen later for evaluation, but not necessarily with the child present. Recently, a mother telephoned after accepting an appointment, stating that her 15-year-old son had agreed to come only if his father, whom he hated, did not come. This was blatant manip-ulation by the child or mother, or both, since the father was living in the home and willing to participate. However, the terms were accepted by the psychiatrist, with the understanding that the father would be included later. A colleague reported that he once had a commune child brought for a first visit by seven adults. We have not had this experience.

In many clinics, the initial family interview is conducted by the multidisciplinary team. This procedure is not feasible in most solo practices, and it does seem that the routine use of the team should be critically reevaluated in view of serious staff shortages and high costs. Including other professionals is an excellent teaching method for trainees and new staff. It may also be justified when there is a good possibility that other professionals will continue with the family in significant di-agnostic or treatment roles. However, it seems doubtful that the cost of routine use of the team interview could be justified in terms of direct benefit to the patient.

At first, these family interviews were very time-consuming for me, but, currently, 1 hour only is reserved for the initial visit. In multidisciplinary clinics, or when the family must travel long distances, an initial visit of 1½ to 2 hours consisting of both group and individual interviews is appropriate. The examiner introduces himself to the family in the waiting area. They are told we will all meet together first, after which there will be some individual discussions, as time permits. They are directed to the office and permitted to choose their seats. The office is comfortable and attractive, but large and utilitarian enough to serve as a therapy place for all but the messiest and most aggressive play activities.

---

*Foster parents are distinguished from adoptive parents in that the latter have been legally established as the true and permanent parents of the child, whereas foster parents usually have a more temporary custodial relationship.

DIAGNOSTIC AND THERAPY CONTRACTS

The interviewer explains that he will be meeting with the family in a series of appointments over the next few weeks, sometimes as a family group but most of the time for individual or private interviews. In this way it will be possible to learn about their problems and come to know them as individuals and as a family. When the doctor has some conclusions, we will meet together again, and he will share his ideas about the difficulties and the procedures he believes will help them. At this point, there is a brief pause and eye contact is made with each person, encouraging questions or comments.

Before any therapy contract can be made, it is essential to reach a consensus on the nature of the problem and the best plan of remediation. We believe the preceding statement of intent constitutes a contract for diagnosis only and in no way commits the family to any treatment plan. The pause is to permit them to ask for clarification or challenge the agreement, but they are not verbally invited to do so. Their silence is taken as consent. If the silence seems strained or painful, they are encouraged to talk about the feelings experienced in making the decision to seek help, getting to the office and, now, actually being there.

If the facial expression of one member, usually the child, shows obvious signs of anger or fear, that impression is conveyed to the individual with the invitation to comment. The response, if any, is accepted and not interpreted in any way. Usually, the child will state feelings in the past tense, referring to the initial reaction upon learning of the plan to see a psychiatrist. The child may be asked whether the feelings or reactions are still the same now that he/she is here. The parents are asked whether they understood the child's reply and are invited to state their own feelings or reactions. One 13-year-old son of devout Jewish parents took the initiative by announcing, "I know what my problem is, Doctor. I have become anti-Semitic." An 8-year-old girl immediately began to cry and said, "I get all scared and have those spells whenever Mommy cries." At this point, the mother began to weep quietly and the father stared nervously at his own shuffling feet. Frequently, a child will verbally, or with silent motions, ask the parents to talk, or one parent may begin by quoting the referring person or stating her own concerns. Silences are never used to force someone to take the initiative. Often, the interviewer will recount briefly what he has been told by the referral source and ask the child what he has been told or ask the parents what they have told the child. Reassurance that it is all right to talk openly in front of each other is freely given, but the wish to remain silent is always respected.

It is impossible to recount all of the directions and forms these sessions take, but some general principles for structuring the interview can be stated. The aims are (1) to promote a free, natural (for this family) discussion among those present; (2) to put them in a cooperative mood for further interviews; and (3) to learn something, but not everything, about their problems and the way they live with each other. The examiner must consciously regulate his own activity-passivity ratio to suit each family. He should actively structure the situation enough to get a clear description of the problems and to prevent irrelevant rambling by dominant persons, scapegoating to the point of cruelty or intolerably painful silences. On the other hand, he must be passive enough to allow spontaneity and to observe the individuals' free responses to him and to each other.

INTERVIEWER NEUTRALITY

Two rules of thumb by which the author abides rather strictly are that (1) the interviewer should try not to take sides or even appear to do so,* and (2) insofar as possible, each family member should be permitted and encouraged to state his or her own views on each issue raised by the examiner's questions or a family member's statements. Early in the session, the family is told that, commonly, family members have different views about many issues and, for the evaluation, it is important that we learn everyone's ideas. They are asked to "hear each other out," even when they strongly disagree with what is being said. They may state that they disagree but are asked not to condemn or punish each other for having expressed an opposing view during the session. In many families, the members are quite

---

*This may be an overstatement in that we often consciously reach out to the child to encourage verbalization. The parents may not want to be in the interview, but they have decided to come and tell their story. However, the child has been brought against his/her will and often has decided in advance to say nothing and to trust no one.

capable of interjecting comments and differing opinions when they know it is safe. For other families, the interviewer must carefully watch facial expressions and use these as cues for interrupting a speaker and calling upon another person to speak. When one person has been notably silent with a blank facial expression, his/her silence may be commented upon and interest expressed in what his/her thoughts might be. If the person cannot talk freely in spite of such encouragement and direction, the silence is merely accepted. The difficulty in communication is mentally noted by the examiner as something to be explored further in individual sessions. Even if such ploys are not successful in promoting open discussion, they clearly acknowledge that views that differ from those of the dominant family member exist and are welcomed by the examiner.

TIMING OF FIRST INTERVIEW

The initial group interview is usually limited to 25 or 30 minutes. In such a short interview, it is sufficient to accomplish only the laying of the ground rules for the ensuing diagnostic sessions and to obtain a reasonably clear picture of the presenting problem and something about the onset and course of symptoms. Any additional data that result from a particularly productive session are considered pure bonus. Sometimes, if the group session is especially fruitful, it may be permitted to continue the entire hour (50 minutes). In such instances, an apology is offered for not having time for any private individual conferences, and assurance is given that these will occur at the next appointment.

If an open discussion cannot be initiated, or even a clear picture of the presenting problem obtained in 20 to 30 minutes, it is useless and sometimes painful to let the session continue. A mental note is made of the communication difficulty. Either the session is terminated or the author shifts to a more structured question-answer-type interview. Such action illustrates an important difference between a diagnostic group interview and family group therapy. In therapy, one would be obligated to identify the communication problem and help the family begin to work on it. In a diagnostic session, one would do better merely to record the finding and defer action until the family is understood better and they are ready to work on that particular problem.

When the group session is terminated, there is never time for three individual sessions. If one person has become and remained visibly upset during the group session, we may say in a tone that seeks family consent, "In the short time left, I would like to have 'X' stay for his/her private session first." Otherwise, the author asks the child to stay for a few private minutes. If one is working with a team, each family member may have a private interview or the parents may be seen conjointly and the child alone. It may be necessary for the team to take a short break to confer briefly without the family. Such a team conference is especially useful for teaching. However, for seasoned professionals who are accustomed to working with each other, the interjection of such conferences may be more disruptive than useful.

The individual interviews immediately after the group meeting are frequently anticlimatic. The interviewer and probably the family may feel "drained." If the preceding session has seemed particularly stressful for the child, those feelings are acknowledged and verbalization is encouraged. The examiner may merely ask general reactions and invite the expression of any ideas that time and circumstances did not permit during the family session. If the child talks or plays willingly, he is permitted to do so while the interviewer observes and gathers data for the mental status assessment. Little effort is made to probe for further information or clarification. It seems better to concentrate on the examiner-child relationship, thereby setting the stage for further interviews. If the child does not talk or play spontaneously we may ask for comments on the problems as stated by the parents: "I'd like to hear your side." If this invitation is declined we take the initiative by switching to a game or a non–emotion-laden topic. It is important for developing the relationship to try to relieve the child of high anxiety or other unpleasant emotions before terminating the interview.

TERMINATING THE FIRST APPOINTMENT

When the appointment time has expired, the child is taken to his parents in the waiting room. The next appointment is made and farewells are exchanged. Should the parents ask for preliminary impressions or direct advice, one should acknowledge their sense of urgency and ask for more examination sessions in the interest of thoroughness and accuracy. You will undermine the entire family's confidence in you if you succumb to such pressure and share undocumented conclusions or give "half-baked" advice. If a parent says, "What do we do until we see you next?" or "Should we do such and such until next time?" look at their faces. If one member has a visible response, ask him/her to respond to the question. If the family is unresponsive, give your honest opinion on whether such action is contraindicated, would be of doubtful value or probably would not be harmful. They can be given permission to do almost anything that the family agrees to give a trial. Whether it works well or not, we can all learn something by discussing the outcome at our next meeting. This clearly establishes the fact that there are no easy pat answers and that solutions will have to be found through concentration and working together.

On rare occasions, something comes up at the last minute that portends possible harm for the child or family and some immediate action is definitely required. These matters cannot be discussed in the waiting area. The family must be taken back to the office to discuss what to do. They may make you late for your next appointment, but so be it.

The beginner clinician is advised not to try to copy my rather rigid time schedule. It took many years of practice before I could limit the initial interview to 1 hour and, even now, I frequently run late. However, the beginner should pay attention to time cost-effectiveness, a matter often ignored in our public-supported training clinics.

IMPORTANT FAMILY OBSERVATIONS

In addition to producing part of the history and providing a unique opportunity to cope with resistances, apprehensions and misconceptions, the group interview provides *in vivo* data on the family functioning and dysfunctioning. In the group session, one can learn about the family's stability, ability to cooperate, capacity for communication, as well as important cultural and social values in a few minutes, whereas it might take several hours to uncover the same data in individual interviews. However, do not expect too much of the family interview. It cannot possibly furnish all of the data needed for a complete psychiatric evaluation of the child and parents.

For obvious reasons, the clinician should never jump to conclusions without double-checking his initial impressions in subsequent examinations of the individuals and the group. Following is a list of elements that are important to learn if we will come to understand the child in his family and the family as a unit. The reader will see that the group interview can quickly provide only some important information relevant to these items.

This list was published in a 1973 G.A.P. report[14] and subsequent clinical experience attests to its validity and usefulness.

1. The nature of the family as a unit (stable, cohesive, divisive, close, distant)
2. The family capacity for cooperation with treatment plans
3. The psychologic-mindedness of members of the family
4. Capacity for communication among family members
5. The degree of mental health or ill health of the family as a unit or in terms of the individual members
6. The role of the child's disorder in the psychic economy of the family (secondary gain, or family misuse of the child's disorder)
7. The relationship of the family to the community (distant, isolated, involved)
8. The subcultural values dominant in the family

CULTURAL AND OTHER VARIABLES

The family interview process described on the preceding pages must be adapted to the interviewer's personality and accommodated to many variables within the family, such as sociocultural factors, intellectual differences, intactness and legal status of the family (divorced parents, foster home, fatherless, motherless, etc.) and the presence of severe handicaps in one or more family members.[15,24] The family intake interview may be appropriate for most families. However, radical changes in the approach are often needed in working with families of different language and cultural backgrounds.

The serious student is urged to read Section Two, "Varieties of Development," in Volume 1 of Noshpitz's *Handbook of Child Psychiatry*.[25] The authors deal with the effects of numerous social variables on the child's development. Their findings can be extrapolated to the family interview situation. Serrano[32] reports that the strong family ties of the Chicano or Mexican-

American family may make family group interviews welcome and rather easy for them. On the other hand, Attneave[3] reports that some American Indian children are strictly taught that speaking up or making eye contact with elders is rude. These latter children may find the author's family interview confounding or even ludicrous. Care must be taken not to interpret cultural differences as signs of psychopathology in the family or its individual members.

Families who share a minority religious or ethnic background are not homogenous groups.[35] The clinician who tries to use his own stereotype to understand the family will mislead himself more often than not. When we do not comprehend the culture of a family, we often cannot discern whether a particular finding or observation merely reflects a cultural difference, is evidence of the family's attempt to integrate itself into its community or is *a priori* evidence of innate psychopathology. When a parent tenaciously holds to a certain belief or type of behavior that seems to impair his child's development, we cannot immediately know whether this is a matter deeply ingrained and vital to the elder's own psychic equilibrium, whether the parent is calloused to his child's needs or whether he or she is just unaware of his own difference from mainstream Americana.

Many mental health professionals in America have had very limited cross-cultural exposure and social interaction with people of different ethnic and religious origins and are thereby limited in their capability for true understanding and empathic comprehension. Efforts to help the child may fail because we cannot establish a workable relationship and simply do not know what to do. Being aware of a deficit in one's background and training may be an initial step in overcoming the problem. It may help for the psychiatrist from middle-class America to view himself as a student and the family as his teacher. Many people are happy to explain their culture if they believe the listener wants to learn rather than pass judgment. Evaluation of these "different" children must be given much more time than usual. The diagnostician must constantly be vigilant lest he offend the family, draw erroneous conclusions or make totally unworkable recommendations.

It has been relatively recent that cultural differences have become a serious concern of professionals other than sociologists and anthropologists. Only in the past few years has the psychiatric literature begun to deal with cultural differences between therapist and patient in instructive rather than judgmental ways. It is true that the clinican will never learn without a strong desire and an open mind. However, these cultural variables are so complex that it takes much more than good intentions and a kind heart to learn to cope with them effectively.

In spite of 35 years in the practice of child psychiatry, I have not had enough cases to offer specific guidelines and illustrations for alterations of the initial approach to the families whose culture and language differ from mine. We are aware that families from other cultures are not referred or do not accept referrals to us and that their drop-out rate, if they do keep an appointment at all, is high. The following adaptations have seemed to help:

1. The appointments are made so that the clinician may offer more or less time than the usual hour.
2. Several, rather than one, family interviews may be needed.
3. The clinician's concern about language, racial or cultural differences impairing his usefulness to the family is brought into the discussion early.
4. Extra effort is needed to dispel mutual distrust and stereotyping.
5. Whenever possible, the assistance of trainees or colleagues from foreign countries or minority Americans should be obtained.*
6. Some clinical centers use indigenous workers from the family's neighborhood, but this rather "new" concept still awaits evaluation.
7. Tenacity and forbearance are important.

Although few specific directions for working with "nonmainstream" American families have been forthcoming from the literature, the popular accusations that middle-class doctors do not care about minorities and minorities do not want their services are both unfair and counterproductive.

---

*With immigrant families the mother is often the least fluent in English because the father is exposed to English-speaking persons at work and the children attend school. It may help to appoint an older child or the father to act as interpreter of your questions to the mother and her replies to you. In individual interviews with a non–English-speaking person a skilled nonfamily interpreter may be essential.

STRESS ON THE EXAMINER

Beginning child psychiatrists often complain of feeling frustrated and tired after their family interviews. Some even suffer headaches or stomachaches. They feel that the stress they experience is greater than what occurs after even very difficult individual interviews. This may be due in part to their having had relatively less experience with group interviews. However, even the experienced psychiatrist can feel excessive personal pressure from some family group sessions.

There are many possible reasons for this stress. The mere fact of the presence of several people and, often, a flood of information from several directions requires intense concentration. It is difficult, perhaps impossible, to do a good interview without some reaching out and personal emotional involvement with the family. The interplay can be fast and the level of everyone's emotions may run high. Transference and countertransference phenomena are complex and, often, there is not time for the evaluator to "tune in" to himself and stay completely comfortable. The things that happen and are said provoke anxiety in the observer, perhaps because they are not comprehensible to him, are personally repugnant or are too similar to some unresolved problem in the interviewer's own current or past family life.

A medical student reported the onset of a significant depression a few days after a "mock" family interview training session in which she had participated. She had volunteered for the training exercise and looked forward to it "as a fun learning experience." She was aware of some marital problems of her own at the time but remembered telling herself that it did not matter. "After all, it was only playacting and I was certain I could pull if off without getting my feelings involved." She became depressed, consulted her instructor and was referred to the student health service for therapy. Later, she recalled what an unpleasant experience her depression had been and how she nearly panicked because final exams were near. However, she philosophically added, "At least it made me seek therapy, something I had probably already put off too long."

Behr[5] reported on the use of simulated interviews as a method of teaching family group principles and technics. He is aware of the participants' stress but does not report any serious untoward sequelae. He believes this is due to a "de-roling" technic that he uses with the students to reduce stress after the sessions.

It is important for the novice to know that he may experience a postinterview stress reaction. He should assure himself of good supervision, a cointerviewer, if possible, and take some time to "mentally unwind" after each session.

SUMMARY

Sometime during a diagnostic evaluation, the examiner should observe the family's interacting together. The author prefers to have the family group interview take place at the initial visit because it reduces distrust and resistance and provides a good opportunity to explain diagnostic procedures to the child and parents together. It shows the child the examiner's attempts to prevent "scapegoating" and helps the family see possible relevant connections of seemingly isolated individual problems to each other.

A brief historical overview of the professional work with parents is presented. Diagnostic and therapeutic interviews are carefully differentiated. By case illustration, my methods are presented, followed by my rationale. Particular attention is paid to cultural phenomena and to the stress effect upon the examiner.

Remember, important information not obtained in the initial interview can usually be learned at subsequent visits. Tolerance for inconclusiveness is necessary.

REFERENCES

1. Ackerman, N.W.: *The Psychodynamics of Family Life.* New York, Basic Books, Inc., 1958, pp. xi–xiii and pp. 351–365.
2. American Academy of Child Psychiatry: *Bibliography of Child Psychiatry and Child Mental Health,* Berlin, I.N. (Ed.). New York, Human Sciences press, 1976, pp. 225–233.
3. Attneave, C.L.: The American Indian Child, Chapter 21 in *Basic Handbook of Child Psychiatry,* Vol. 1, *Development,* Noshpitz, J.D. (Ed.). New York, Basic Books, Inc., 1979, pp. 239–248.
4. Augenbraun, B.: Differential techniques in family interviewing with both parents and preschool child. J. Am. Acad. Child Psychiatry, *5:*721, 1966.
5. Behr, H.L.: Introducing medical students to family therapy using simulated family interviews. Med. Educ., *11:*32, 1977.
6. Beavers, H.R. and Voeller, M.N.: Family models: Comparing and contrasting the systems model. Fam. Process, *22:*85–98, 1983.
7. Brown, S.L.: Diagnosis, clinical management and family interviewing in

childhood and adolescence in *Science and Psychoanalysis,* Vol. 14, Wasserman, J.H. (Ed.). New York, Grune & Stratton, 1969, pp. 188–198.

8. ———: Family interviewing as a basis for clinical management, in *The Family: Evaluation and Treatment,* Hofling, C.K. and Lewis, J.M. (Eds.). New York, Brunner/Mazel, 1980, pp. 122–137.

9. Burdette, James A.: Comprehensive interviewing in the family physician office practice: A suggested technique. Southwestern Med., *51*:124, 1970.

10. Freedman, A.M., Kaplan, H.I., and Sadock, B.J. (Eds.): *Modern Synopsis of Comprehensive Textbook of Psychiatry/II,* 2nd Ed. Baltimore, Williams and Wilkins Co., 1976, pp. 1023–35.

11. Freud, A.: *The Psychoanalytic Treatment of Children.* New York, International Universities Press, 1946.

12. Gaines, T.: Factors influencing a failure to show for a family evaluation. Int. J. Fam. Counseling, *6*:57–61, 1978.

13. Grossman, J.A., Poznauski, E.O., and Banegas, M.E.: Time to study family interactions. J. Psycho-social Nurs., Mental Health Service, *21*:19–23, 1983.

14. Group for the Advancement of Psychiatry: *From Diagnosis to Treatment: An Approach to Treatment Planning for the Emotionally Disturbed Child, Report No. 87.* New York, 1973.

15. ———: *The Case History Method in the Study of Family Process, Report No. 76.* New York, 1970, pp. 251–261.

16. ———: *The Field of Family Therapy, Report No. 78.* New York, 1970, pp. 572–580.

17. Howells, J.G.: Principles of Family Therapy. New York, Brunner/Mazel, 1975, pp. 175–250.

18. Kanner, L.: *Child Psychiatry,* 2nd Ed. Springfield, Ill., Charles C Thomas, Publisher, 1948, pp. 3–16 and 244–247.

19. Klein, M.: *The Psychoanalysis of Children.* New York, Grove Press, 1932.

20. Krill, D.F.: Family interviewing as an intake diagnostic method. Soc. Work, *13*:56, 1968.

21. Malone, C.A.: Child psychiatry and family therapy: An overview. J. Am. Acad. Child Psychiatry, *18*:4, 1979.

22. McDermott, J.F., Jr.: Family therapy in child psychiatry. J. Am. Acad. Child Psychiatry, *18*:1, 1979.

23. Moore, M.U.: *Contributions of Orthopsychiatry to Family Casework, in Orthopsychiatry: Retrospect and Prospect,* Lowery, L.G. and Sloane, V. (Eds.). New York, American Orthopsychiatric Association, Inc., 1948, pp. 310–323.

24. Noshpitz, J.D. (Ed.): *Basic Handbook of Child Psychiatry,* Vol. 1, *Development.* New York, Basic Books, Inc., 1979, pp. 239–485.

25. Olson, D., Sprenkl, B., and Russell, C.: Circumplex model of marital and family systems. Fam. Proc., *18*:29–44, 1979.

26. Perlmutter, R.A., and Jones, J.E.: Assessment of families in psychiatric emergencies. Am. J. Orthopsychiatry, *55*:131–139, 1985.

27. Roberts, C.S., and Feetham, S.L.: Assessing family functioning across three areas of relationships. Nurs. Res., *31*:231–235, 1982.

28. Rosenfelt, A., and Newberger, E.H.: Compassion versus control. J.A.M.A., *237*:2086–2088, 1977.

29. Ruhrah, G.: *Pediatrics of the Past.* New York, Paul B. Hoeber, Inc., 1925.

30. Sager, C., Masters, Y., Ronall, R., and Normand, J.: Selection and engagement of patients in family therapy. Am. J. Orthopsychiatry, *38*:715–723, 1968.

31. Selvini-Palazzoli, M., Boscolo, L., Cecchin, G., and Prata, G.: Hypothesizing—circularity—neutrality: Three guidelines for the conductor of the session. Fam. Proc., *19*:3–13, 1980.

32. Serrano, A.C., and Castillo, F.G.: The Chicano child and his family, Chapter

23 in *Basic Handbook of Child Psychiatry*, Vol. 1, *Development*. Noshpitz, J.D. (Ed.). New York, Basic Books, Inc., 1979, pp. 624–630.

33. Sigal, J.: A simple dynamic model for family diagnostic interviewing. Can. Psychiatr. Assoc. J., *16*:87, 1971.

34. Simmons, J.E.: Parent treatability: What is it? J. Am. Acad. Child Psychiatry, *20*:4, 1981.

35. Spurlock, J., and Lawrence, L.E.: The Black child, Chapter 22 in *Basic Handbook of Child Psychiatry*, Vol. 1, *Development*. Noshpitz, J.D. (Ed.). New York, Basic Books, Inc., 1979, pp. 248–257.

36. Teisman, M.W.: Convening strategies in family therapy. Fam. Proc., *19*:393–400, 1980.

37. Tyler, E.A., Truumaa, A., and Henshaw, P.: Family group intake by a child guidance clinical team. Arch. Gen. Psychiatry, *6*:214, 1962.

38. Vaughn, C., and Leff, J.: The measurement of expressed emotion in the families of psychiatric patients. Br. J. Soc. Clin. Psych., *15*:157, 1976.

39. Viaro, M., and Leonardi, P.: Getting and giving information: Analysis of a family interview strategy. Fam. Proc., *22*:27–42, 1983.

40. Walker, L.G., Thomson, N., and Lindsay, W.R.: Assessing family relationships: A multimethod, multisituational approach. Br. J. Psychiatry, *144*:387–394, 1981.

41. Webster-Stratton, C.: Comparison of abusive and nonabusive families with conduct disordered children. Am. J. Orthopsychiatry, *55*:59–69, 1985.

42. Wells, C.F., and Rabiner, E.L.: The conjoint family diagnostic interview and the family index of tension. Fam. Proc., *12*:127, 1973.

43. Zimmerman, G.: Adolescents in crisis: The usefulness of family interview. Am. J. Psychiatry, *128*:1025, 1972.

3

INDIVIDUAL INTERVIEWS
WITH THE CHILD

The information to be obtained during the child's examination is the same as that needed for the mental status examination of adults: e.g., orientation, affect, stream of thought, fantasies, ambitions, concept of self, interpersonal relations, ideals, mannerisms, and so on. The methods of obtaining these data depend very much upon the age and nature of the child, the training and personality of the examiner, and the setting in which the examination takes place. The psychiatric examination is incomplete until sufficient material is obtained to write a complete mental status report. This is time-consuming and takes several interviews.

EQUIPMENT FOR THE INTERVIEW ROOM

In general, a greater number of possible activities are needed for ongoing psychotherapy than for diagnostic interviews. A wide variety of activities, as well as the opportunity to do things and to do them together with the therapist, are often essential in therapy. In our clinic we maintain two traditional playrooms that any staff member may schedule for specific hours when use of his own office-playroom might be impractical.

The following items may be found in either or both of these rooms: pullman kitchenette for cooking and baking; sinks for water play; space for large-muscle activities; a variety of art materials such as clay, paints, and crayons; tools and woodworking bench; building blocks; baby dolls; miniature-life dolls; puppets; toy soldiers and guns; furnished dollhouse; assorted trains, trucks, cars, and planes; sandbox; models for assembly; and assorted table games. The exact content of the rooms varies somewhat from time to time, depending upon the fads or convictions of the staff. So far as possible, most of these materials are kept in cupboards with sliding doors to facilitate periodic cleaning of the room and to give the therapist some control over the amount and kind of stimuli presented to a particular child. A family of dolls with realistic genitals is available to be signed out when needed.

It may be impractical for the lone practitioner to maintain such a variety of equipment for a comparatively smaller number of patients. Although the items noted here are often, but not always, needed for continuing child psychotherapy, we have found the following quite adequate for diagnostic interviews and much of our therapy in the playroom-office combination: some creative art materials, some toys for aggressive fantasy play, a few action toys (trucks or cars), doll or puppets for depicting interaction and personal projection, and some table games to be used for interaction with the examiner and to permit evasion of or relief from emotion-laden activities. Variations can and should be made from this baseline as the clinician finds additions or alterations that enhance the productivity of the youngsters seen in diagnosis and therapy.

Besides the playroom and adequately equipped offices, the child psychiatrist finds many other readily available settings that can be used. Children's general distaste for close confinement and the fact that they are less inhibited about personal matters than adults make it permissible to take young patients out of the playroom or office at times. The elevator and the basement of a building are most interesting and stimulating. The street, the local playground, the drugstore soda fountain, the construction projects in the next block, and many other areas can be considered part of the child psychiatrists' interviewing equipment.

The decision to take a child outside the office or playroom has its pitfalls. Most people learn at a very early age that discomfort in social situations is relieved by either changing the subject of conversation or moving about, preferably to a different setting. If the examiner becomes anxious for any one of a variety of reasons, she may take the child "out to play" to "help him relate better." Psychiatrists are so accustomed to talking about such topics as sex, violence, or sadness that we don't feel uncomfortable with the verbal child, no matter what she says. However, symbolic play of these emotions, refusal to say or do anything, or gestures and words that are too personally directed may provoke us to take the child out of the examining room without realizing it is our own and not the child's discomfort that is being handled. A decision or action by the examiner is correct if it facilitates the purpose of the hour. Sometimes we cannot be sure about the correct action until we have tried it. When a child is taken out for play during a diagnostic exam, we must ask ourselves whether we learned anything about the child. If not, then we would have done well to have remained in the office. We tread a narrow line here. It would be cruel to confine a child to the office if he is overwhelmed with his own thoughts and fears. On the other hand we do the child no favor if we engage her in activities that prevent her from ever revealing herself.

TRAINING AND PERSONALITY OF THE PSYCHIATRIST

The formal training requirements and examination procedures necessary to obtain recognition as a specialist in child psychiatry are outlined by the Subcommittee on Child Psychiatry of American Board of Psychiatry and Neurology, Inc.[2] These include fulfillment of all the training and licensing requirements for general medical practice, training and certification in general psychiatry, and finally special training and certification in child psychiatry. Hence from a pragmatic standpoint the kind of person who becomes a child psychiatrist is predetermined by various admissions officers or the admissions committees of colleges, medical schools, general psychiatric residency training programs, child psychiatry training programs, the American Board of Psychiatry and Neurology, and the organization's Subcommittee on Child Psychiatry. Finally, a local medical society, a state medical licensing board, the board of directors of a community clinic, and parents will have some say in determining the sort of person who will be the psychiatrist for any particular child.

Whether or not the long, arduous, and rather cumbersome selection process that has evolved really provides us with those persons from the total population who are best suited to fulfill a specific mental health need for the next generation may be debated—in fact, is rather hotly debated at times in some circles. It can be said with certainty that each selecting authority numerically reduces the field of choice for the next higher authority. No doubt some persons are kept out of the profession who would have much to offer, and others with comparatively little potential slip through this screening network. We can only hope that the numbers in each of these categories are small. If so, this is indeed fortuitous, since few of these selecting bodies have the specific selection of someone to care for mentally ill children as their primary concern.

Every young man or woman who considers entering the profession should give serious thoughts to her/his own suitability. The reader knows that interest and motivation are primary factors that have many unconscious determinants. These and other unconscious elements of one's own personality may serve us well or poorly in future work with children. The fact that children, especially sick ones, create an emotional impact upon the adult makes it essential that the child psychiatrist have considerable insight into his/her own behavior. In addition to helping the resident trainee accumulate knowledge and clinical skills, a major goal of many, perhaps most, preceptors is to help the resident develop useful insight into his own emotional responses to patients.

In the 1940s and 1950s, many preceptors insisted upon personal psychoanalysis for their child psychiatry candidates as means of providing this insight. Even though some still hold to this tenet, it has appeared to many as neither entirely practical nor at times particularly effective. One might say the same for child psychiatrists as can be said for parents: for many, personal psychotherapy is essential to reach even a modicum of success as either a parent or a child therapist; for others, effective functioning can be greatly enhanced by therapy. Certainly the matter deserves serious consideration by all trainees and supervisors. At this time, however, no absolute rules about personal analysis seem possible. The child psychiatrists of this country serve in a variety of functions—as therapists, diagnosticians, researchers, administrators, and child care consultants, to name a few. No one can ever be the epitome of perfection in all these areas. Candidates should use their own conscience and the observations of preceptors to determine whether their daily work is socially and professionally effective and, if not, to determine whether personal therapy is the answer.

Preparation for work in child psychoanalysis is beyond the scope of this monograph. The interested reader may be directed to sources of information regarding training in child psychoanalysis by the American Psychoanalytic Association or by a psychoanalytic institute in a specific geographical area.

AGE AND NATURE OF THE CHILD

Of the three variables in the diagnostic interview—the examination setting, the examiner, and the patient—the most important is the patient. It would take many volumes to discuss each age level and the many behavioral variations related to age. Here, however, a few general comments about children as psychiatric patients are in order.

There is great danger of skewing all the information if one is preoccupied too early with delineating normal and abnormal behavior. The assessment of normality or abnormality is discussed in the next section. During the examination itself, the emphasis should be upon learning to know the child as thoroughly as possible without jumping to conclusions or making value judgments.

Great allowances must be made for children's attitudes toward the examiner and the examination. Many children appear resistive and negative when brought to the psychiatrist's office. From the child's standpoint these attitudes are completely justified.[5] The child psychiatric patient is similar to the committed adult patient in that usually she had no part in the decision to seek professional help and has been brought for the examination against her will. Past experience may well have proved that all adults are in collusion, and she feels that the examiner is no exception. Certainly the children know that there was some communication between the examiner and the parents in order to arrange the appointment "behind her back," and since the parents are paying the fee it is only natural that the psychiatrist's alliance would be with them. They believe that adults really have little interest in understanding children except for nefarious purposes. Commonly, whether the child admits it or not, he firmly believes that the examination will give positive proof of innate badness and will justify further punishment from the parents.

A language barrier can present problems between the physician and the patient. Adolescents and certain ethnic groups often use colloquialisms and dialects in a conscious attempt to maintain their privacy from the conventional world. Younger children are still developing from primary process thinking to

secondary process thinking. Their ability to use abstract concepts and to express feelings and ideas at a verbal level is often
limited. These limitations provide one reason why play is so
essential to child diagnosis and therapy. The child can express
herself in action much more easily than with words.

Adults usually have considerable difficulty in comprehending the play language of children. The chapter in Erikson's
book[4] entitled "Toys and Reasons" is strongly recommended
to the student of child psychiatry. Erikson reminds us that, to
the adult, play means recreation or respite from work. On the
other hand, play is a principal occupation of childhood and
has much more personal significance than merely a relief from
the workaday world. Play activity usually has a common meaning for a group of children of similar age and background. It
will also have a unique meaning for any individual within the
group. To comprehend the unique meaning, one must not only
observe the play's content and form, but also have the child
tell accompanying fantasies and reveal the affect associated
with the play. Erikson believes that much of the unique meaning
of play is concerned with the child's efforts to master himself,
his/her own body and body sensations, and the anxiety stimulated by the world and events around. Through play the child
learns to master reality by experiment and planning. Erikson
points out that it is a definite human trait at any age to deal
with experience by creating model situations. He quotes William Blake: "The child's toys and the old man's reasons are the
fruit of the two seasons."

For obvious reasons the dissocial or delinquent child can be
expected to be considerably more resistant to the examination
than the average child. Aichhorn[1] explains that such children,
particularly those lacking in neurotic guilt over their behavior,
approach all adults with a negative transference of distrust and
hostility. The adult must be able to take the child's part and
agree with the behavior under the circumstances. When these
children boldly lie or maintain stoic silence, the examiner
should control her irritation and the usual adult impulse to
expose the culprit's hostility and untruthfulness. Sometimes
distrust can be attacked directly by agreeing that it is dangerous
to confide in strange adults but reminding the patient that some
subjects can be mutually discussed without this danger. Aichhorn lets the child know that he is not fooled by him, but neither
is he angry over these justifiable attempts at trickery. To make

this point he sometimes uses gentle, transparent sarcasm in the form of spoofing the child by telling grosser lies.

Frank, nonjudgmental discussion of the child's delinquent actions can disarm him and help him confide to you his concept of the outer limits of right and wrong. No matter how far he is from the social average, each individual has some line or point beyond which he considers behavior to be wrong. Some homely examples are the common belief that it is all right to steal small amounts, but not large ones, or that it is not particularly reprehensible to pilfer from the government or large corporations, but it is serious to appropriate a neighbor's possessions. The following case illustrates the use of frank, open discussion as a means of ascertaining the standards that have been internalized by the patient.

> Jack, an 11-year-old, had been placed in juvenile detention for stealing and vandalism, and his court worker had requested a psychiatric evaluation. After a brief general conversation, the subject of his detention came up. Jack quickly professed his innocence and the fact that he was implicated by others on purely circumstantial evidence.
>
> E: I know that but tell me—under ordinary circumstances what do you like to steal the most?
>
> JACK: Oh, anything, just anything.
>
> E: What's the most you've ever really been able to get away with?
>
> J: Oh, I guess a bicycle worth about twenty bucks. Oh, yea, I got fifteen dollars from my uncle Harry's dresser once.
>
> E: See my fountain pen? Would you steal that?
>
> J: No, not unless I was sure I could get a running start on you.
>
> E: How come they claim it's always wrong to steal from banks and stores when those places got lots of money?
>
> J: Cause you will get sent to prison for it. (This last comment portrays reliance upon external controls as a major deterrent to antisocial behavior.
>
> After some additional conversation on other topics, the matter of sex was approached. Jack volunteered that he knew everything about that.)
>
> E: How old were you when you first had sex with a girl?
>
> J: It was last year when I was 10.
>
> E: Was she your girl friend?
>
> J: Nah, she was my cousin.
>
> E: What happened?
>
> J: My aunt caught us.
>
> E: What happened?
>
> J: She told my mother.
>
> E: What happened?
>
> J: My mother said you ain't supposed to do that with your relations.

It is essential to remember that the psychiatrist is not assigned the task of extracting a confession. The task is to obtain a professional opinion of the overall functioning of the patient. Therefore, questions are not designed to learn whether or not an act has been committed. One may ask questions as if the fact of their occurrence had already been settled. (As here, the psychiatrist asked when not whether the child had had sex.) The child is then free to deny the implied allegations, or he may decide that, since guilt or innocence is not an issue, he can readily reveal the details. Some delinquents will enjoy responding to the question "How did you happen to get caught?" but are made angry by questions about why or whether a certain act was committed.

STRUCTURING THE INTERVIEW SITUATION

Werkman,[9] Beiser,[3] Martin,[7] and many others have described their interview approaches, which are varying combinations of play and conversation. Manipulating the child's play according to some memorized structured interview procedure is likely to suppress the child's spontaneity. On the other hand, mere passive observations of the child's play without eliciting any verbal associations may leave the examiner confused as to the specific significance of the child's activities.

This author uses a moderately active conversational method of interview in an office-playroom. In general, children less than 10 or 11 years of age are most comfortable and productive when using the play materials, and older children readily respond to the conversational method of examination. Some 14- or 15-year-olds, however, spontaneously use the toys, usually as a tension-relieving device. On the other hand, some 6- or 7-year-olds, unable to use the play materials, are able to indulge in direct conversation about themselves and the significant events or people in their lives.

As stated previously, children should not be encouraged to "do" something or be forced to play. If they appear interested, they can be told that they may use any of the things in the room. If they play spontaneously, questions may be interjected from time to time to clarify the action and thinking. If they seem content to sit and talk, let them do so. Should they become increasingly anxious in the examination instead of more spontaneous, they may be taken out for a walk or a treat or urged to play.

There should be an abundance of time for any interview. The examiner's activity-passivity ratio must be geared to a level that promotes the child's productivity, and the approach has to be altered considerably from child to child. The patient should be given ample opportunity to be spontaneous, keeping in mind that prolonged silences can be anxiety-provoking to many children. On one occasion after a one-way-vision-room demonstration, a group of medical students asked whether the examiner was purposely using silence to provoke and upset the patient. The examiner had not been aware that the patient was particularly anxious. Whether the child was unduly distressed by the silence or not remains uncertain, but the medical students had reacted negatively to it. It has been our observation that medical students push and talk too much in interviews. Psychiatrists are likely to err on the side of overusing silence.

The word *why* should be avoided as much as possible. "Why?" often sounds too much like an accusation or implies that the situation is wrong and needs justification. If the child knew the answer, she probably would not need professional help. Children have been negatively conditioned by adult use of the word *why*. Often a parent asks, "Why did you do it?" or "Why didn't you do such and such?" During a play situation the question "Why did doll 'A' run out of the house?" may disrupt the play. Putting the question as "What was doll 'A' thinking about when she/he ran out of the house?" may facilitate the child's associations. Asking the patient why he or she wishes to be a firefighter or police officer or a nurse when grown up implies that he must justify his decision. It is better to ask what police officers or nurses do that the child finds particularly interesting or fun. Instead of asking why a particular event in her history occurred, she can be asked "Where were you and what were all the people doing just before that happened? How were you feeling? How did it make you feel afterward?" The following is a list of 10 broad, general topics around which an interview may be loosely structured.

1. Reasons for coming or being brought for the examination
2. Recreation and interests
3. Social, cultural, and ethnic group and the child's harmony with it
4. Peer relationships
5. Plans for the future
6. Family relationship
7. Additional discussion of the presenting problem

8. General health (psychophysiologic status)
9. Fantasies and fears
10. Social awareness

As mentioned previously, the child often initiates the interview by acting out a problem or illustrating some significant aspect of her interpersonal relations. She may talk directly about these subjects or use symbols and play. During the course of several interviews, some children spontaneously give considerable information on each of the foregoing topics. Others spontaneously include most of the items, and with relatively few questions the examiner can obtain information on subjects that did not come up spontaneously. Still other children require a considerable amount of activity by the examiner.

The topics may be covered in any order that seems natural. Frequently it helps to ask questions indirectly or buffer them with comments such as "Some kids have told me they expected the clinic to be a lot different than it is." "A little girl/boy told me the other day that she had lots of trouble with her brothers and sisters. Have you ever known anyone who felt like that?" Teachers, playmates, or parents may be substituted in the question for brothers and sisters. Whenever possible, the open-end type of question is used. If questions meet with silence, the child is permitted to remain silent or pursue other activities. I often tell children that they may say "I don't know" if they truly don't know the answer to a question, but if they know the answer and don't want to say it they may say "I don't want to talk about that." Some children can't believe I honestly give permission to openly refuse to talk.

Reasons for Coming or Being Brought for the Examination

Ask what the child has been told and what he thought the purpose was. Inquire about feelings about the visit. If he has been told nothing or does not know, suggest that he guess, or that he guess why others might come to see the physician. He can be reassured if he expresses fear about the visit. The examiner should identify herself and her reasons for interest in the child. If you know that there is particularly severe antagonism between the child and the parents, it is occasionally helpful to reveal this knowledge to the child and invite him to tell his side of the story. This approach and these questions were discussed in the section on the initial interview. However, when the child is unwilling to discuss problems, it is useless to try to probe deeply until you are comfortable together, possibly not until the second or third interview.

Recreation and Interests

When the child spontaneously reveals some of her special talents or interests, it is an easy matter to gain considerable information by polite questions about details. If she gives you no clues, she can be asked directly about her hobbies or the kinds of activities she thinks are particularly fun. The interview is helped by talking about nonproblem areas or areas of success, and considerable information about the child's abilities and interests or lack of them, compared with her age group, can be learned. On these topics one should be able to see a child at her best and note her organization of thinking, her stream of thought, and her attention span and perhaps even obtain clues to her intellectual capabilities.

Social, Cultural, and Ethnic Group and the Child's Harmony with It

Inquiries may be made about school, church, and the neighborhood. What does he like best about these places, and what does he like least? What are the people like whom he finds there? What do his parents say about these places? Ask what is most troublesome in school: the teachers, the studies, or the other children? Has he ever changed schools, or would he like to? What kinds of things are or would be different at the other school?

When the examiner's race, culture, social status or accent differs from the child's or the family's the examiner should bring up the matter for discussion if the child has not spontaneously done so in the first two interviews. We are easily aware of the child's difference from us but are inclined to ignore (repress) our differences from her. It is always the other person who has the "funny accent," has the "strange beliefs" or acts as if his difference is "normal" and easily accepted. One can say to the child "Did you notice we pronounce (say) the same words differently? have different color skins? use words the other one never heard before?" (Identify whatever the most obvious "difference" is.) "Did that surprise you when we first met? What did that make you think and feel when you first noticed our difference?" With adolescents be more explicit. "Have you had previous experience with women doctors? A Chinese doctor? A Black doctor? Is my accent hard to understand? Please ask me to repeat if you don't understand me."

The examiner can continue, "Have you known other people like me in the movies or on TV, at school or other places?" The examiner can gently explore the child's reactions to those other people and situations, gradually bringing the discussion around to the here and now. "How does our difference(s) affect your feelings about coming to see me? Does my (difference—name it) ever get you upset, scared, confused, or mad or make you feel like not coming back?" If the child can identify negative feelings, it is proper to explore ways to make the visits less problematic. Many, perhaps most, children cannot or will not discuss feelings stemming from differences. However, the mere fact of bringing up such matters as possible problems may relieve much of the child's discomfort and resistance. At the very least, an interchange such as the one described assures the child he can talk about these matters any time he notices them.

Some examiners make a concerted effort to avoid their own colloquialisms; use only the simplest, shortest words, and even copy the accent and jargon of the patient. Noble as the motives might be, it is impossible to disguise or "whitewash" speaking and behavioral mannerisms of a lifetime completely. Some well-trained actors can do this convincingly, especially on the stage or screen openly designated as a place for playacting. Off-stage in real life, there is the risk of appearing condescending, pedantic, insincere or just plain silly. It is probably better to tell the child that our differences may make it hard to talk to and understand each other. When we do not understand, both of us (child and doctor) have the right to ask the other to explain what she is saying or what she means.

There may be many more subtle cultural differences that do not become obvious until therapy is well under way. Such factors cannot be predicted and, therefore, must be handled when they appear, in the context of the current therapy situation.

The preceding suggestions are offered only as methods that may facilitate the diagnostic process, put the patient and doctor more at ease with each other and increase the examiner's understanding of the patient. The beginner must remember that feelings, confusion and misunderstandings stemming from cultural, ethnic, racial or religious differences are never really resolved during the diagnostic process. These matters become a part of ongoing therapy and will recur again and again during any long-term therapeutic endeavor.

Peer Relationships

Knowledge of peer relationships as the child sees them gives considerable information about the capacity to make meaningful interhuman relations and identifications, the degree of social awareness, and the level of independence. Does he have one friend or a few best friends, or does he claim social relations with nearly everyone? What are the depth and nature of these close relationships, if they exist? Do they tell each other secrets? How frequently are they in contact? What kinds of activities do they do together, and how do they settle their disagreements? Who are some of the kids he doesn't like or who do not like him? What kind of differences do they have? Inquiries about clubs and team memberships are appropriate, and the child should be encouraged to compare himself with others in his age group as to relative size, intelligence, leadership, and so on.

Plans for the Future

When asked what they would like to be when they grow up, most children appear embarrassed and say that they do not know yet. They can be reassured that you know the final decision cannot be made at this time. Yet almost all of us think of a number of things from time to time that we would like to be, even though we change our minds. What are some of the things that she has considered? What do people of that vocation do? Which of these activities have any special appeal? Some little girls say that they would enjoy being nurses because they help sick children; others believe that it would be fun because nurses get to give shots. Some children see police officers as maintaining law and order, and others admire them as people who have legal sanction to shoot other people.

After growing up and finding work, does the child think that he will marry? Has the potential partner already been chosen? What does he think he would like best about being married, and what least? Would he like to have children of his own? How many? Would he rather have boys or girls, and what are the relative advantages? What has he been told about where babies come from and how they got there?

Family Relationships

Children should be encouraged to tell about the pleasant family relationships and the fun they have both as a group and individually with siblings, as well as with the mother and father separately. They can then be asked about what kinds of things might make them angry with each other. How do the family members express their anger, and with whom are they most often angry? When someone is angry, how does the patient and how do the parents react to this? How much do they know about their parents' vocations, and how do they feel about their work?

Very young patients may be presented with a simple drawing of a mother and a child that the examiner has sketched. The drawing should be neutral about the child's sex. The patient is then asked to describe what he sees. He will usually give the child the same sex as his own. He can then be asked the age of the child and about relations between mother and child. He can be asked what the child does to make his mother happy or angry and what the mother does when she experiences these feelings. What kinds of things does the mother do that make the child particularly happy or angry? What does the child do when he experiences these feelings? The same sketch may be used for the father. In the anger situation, most children describe some form of withdrawal as their usual response. They should then be asked what they felt like doing. Do they think of attacking? or running away? Have they ever done so? Suicidal and homicidal impulses should also be questioned.

> Ian was a 9-year-old boy who was referred by the mother's psychotherapist. Ian's parents had separated 3½ months ago and were planning a divorce. Mother was 34 years old. Father was 30. They had been married for 10 years. "Ian has become extremely upset and uncontrollable. In response to minor frustration, he goes into violent rages. He swears, breaks things, kicks his mother, throws rocks at his siblings and runs away." The mother could not control him. She was becoming exhausted and feared he might harm himself or others. Mother and her therapist wondered whether Ian should be hospitalized for his own protection as well as to give mother some relief.
>
> On the first three diagnostic visits Ian was seen with both of his parents and also had two half-hour sessions alone with the examiner. During individual interviews, Ian played vigorously but not destructively with the dart game and then played quietly with some puzzles. Part of the time he spontaneously sat and talked. He described his "fits" of anger and the fact that both he and his mother want father to come back. He had once shouted that he wanted to kill himself, but he didn't mean it. He was just mad at his mother. His memory was poor. He could not

remember details, gave no information that had not already been given by his parents and could not or would not expand on his subjective feelings.

At the fourth visit, Ian was told that we would have 45 minutes alone and he would not have to share the time with his parents. He seemed pleased. He entered the room, sat in a chair and ignored the toys. The following interchange took place:

IAN: Mother wants me to tell you about Sunday.

EXAMINER: Do you want to tell me about it?

I: No.

E: You know I'd like to hear about it, but you don't have to tell me if you don't want to.

I (with an embarrassed grin): I had another one of my "fits." I threw a rock at Brian (7-year-old brother). He keeps bothering me. He jumps on me and tries to kiss me and nobody does anything about it. He yells when I am on the telephone. I want Mom to punish Brian, but she won't.

E: You must wonder why Mother doesn't punish him?

I: Yeah. It seems like he's too good and I'm always getting punished. He does all this stuff and she just says, "Stop it, Brian." She punishes me for the same things.

E: Does that make you feel she likes him better?

I: Yeah.

E: How do you feel then?

I: Sad.

E: What else do you feel?

I: Mad (silence).

E: You must wonder why she treats him better?

I: Yeah. I guess it's cause he's younger. It's been like that ever since I was 5, when I started the fits. I went to a psychiatrist when I was 6 (silence). Sometimes I wish Mom was gone. Sometimes I wish they were both gone. I want Dad to come home but sometimes I'm glad he's gone.

E: Do you love them?

I: Yes (silence). It seems like he's divorcing us (brother and Ian) more than Mom.

E: What do you mean?

I: It seemed he left because of us kids.

E: You look pretty sad about all this.

I: Yeah. I really do think about killing myself. I think about stabbing myself or starting up the car.

E: Starting up the car?

I: You know—the exhaust fumes. That will get you fast.

E: What has kept you from killing yourself?

I: The Bible says you'll go down there (points to the ground) if you commit suicide. I don't think I believe the Bible (silence). No one should want to kill himself. That's just stupid.

E: When you're feeling very bad, what helps?

I: Nothing (silence). I just settle down myself. I stop the fit.

E: How do you feel then?

I: Sort of sad I threw the fit, but I feel better. I got it all out but it makes matters worse (brief silence). Some people have heart attacks if they hold it inside.

E: Do you worry about having a heart attack?

I: Aren't I too young to get a heart attack?

E: I'm interested in what you said about Dad leaving because of you kids.

I: I'm pretty sure the divorce is mostly my fault. Brian and I fight all the time and get Mom all upset.

E: I know your Mom and Dad don't like it when you and your brother fight, and most kids usually think they have caused their parents' divorce. However, I have talked to them (the parents) and I know they have lots of problems and fights that don't even have anything to do with you and Brian.

I: Well, it seems Mother and Dad are hurting us more than anyone, 'cause we're such brats (brief silence).

Ian then challenged the examiner to a game of darts. He played quietly and without enthusiasm. He did not talk about his parents or the divorce anymore but told a rather long, involved story about his cousins who are real mean and who got arrested for vandalizing the neighbor's barn.

At the first interview the parents had been given some suggestions for coping with Ian's outbursts. The father stated categorically that he planned to terminate the marriage and that his work made it impossible for him to "come running" each time Ian threw a fit. The examiner commented that it looked as if the mother would have to calm down Ian as best she could when he had a temper outburst. He (the examiner) asked the mother whether she would be willing to defer hospitalization until we had tried some of the ideas discussed.

There was a lessening of the intensity and frequency of Ian's outbursts over the next few weeks. However, after the fourth visit in which be blamed himself for the divorce, Ian's tantrums dramatically stopped, as did his misbehavior on the school bus. (It should be noted that during these few weeks the school principal had been very helpful in consoling, controlling and counseling Ian when he had problems on the bus or playground.)

On the basis of his symptoms one could justify a descriptive diagnosis of Conduct Disorder, Socialized, Aggressive. He also fulfilled many of the criteria for Dysthymic Disorder. Many of his symptoms were provoked or precipitated by his chaotic home situation. His mother also had suffered episodes of depression since her early teens. Her personality was marked by extreme passive dependency with some antisocial trends. She was quite unable to provide structure and consistent discipline for Ian and his younger brother since the father left. She had voluntarily placed two older children with her sister some time before this marriage. These children were from a previous marriage and were now 15 and 16 years of age. The current husband seemed interested in the boys and said he felt guilty about leaving them, but he could not cope with his wife's emotional vicissitudes.

Placement of Ian outside his home was deferred because of his apparent deep attachment to both his parents and the possibility of further skewing his personality development. A trial of individual psychotherapy for Ian along with intensive counseling of the parents was recommended. The goals for the parents were not to save the marriage, but to try to teach the mother more effective home discipline and to counsel both parents on how to avoid getting Ian caught in the middle of their conflicts. Therapy was scheduled weekly, with parents' alternating bringing him and having their own counseling session. The situation remained stormy and tenuous with frequent "emergency" sessions between the scheduled times. Antidepressant medication for Ian was considered, but not used, since he made definite and fairly rapid improvement. The mother was receiving antidepressant medication from her therapist.

By the end of the school semester Ian's temper outbursts had completely abated and he was doing well in school again. His improvement cannot be said to be due entirely to the psychotherapy for by this time the divorce was final and matters of support, custody and visitation were being worked out. Therapy sessions were spaced out, and he was discharged from treatment 9 months after the first diagnostic session.

Ian is now 14 years old. In a recent follow-up, the mother reported that she is no longer in therapy. She began working a few months after the divorce and Ian began skipping school. Mother remarried and her present husband does not like children. He is a firm disciplinarian. Also Ian and his younger brother do not get along well. Ian asked to live with his father and the latter's girlfriend and was permitted to do so even though the mother suspected the father used drugs and alcohol. Last year Ian went to the police station and reported the father and girlfriend for using drugs. Mother was uncertain of the details; at about that time he threatened suicide again, but "nothing came of it."

Ian does not use drugs and has not been in trouble at school or in the community. His grades vary from passing to A's. He visits his mother every other weekend and is in her home frequently in between regular visitation. He gets along with his current stepfather and she believes she has a good relationship with him.

Additional Discussion of the Presenting Problem

Even though the child may have been willing to discuss the presenting symptoms during the initial phases of the first interview, it is always a good idea to review problem areas directly with him in some detail after the relationship has been established. He can be asked whether they seem to be getting worse or better and how worried about them he might be. Ask what he thinks might help. Inquiry can be made about previous examiners or therapists, if there have been any, and his concept of ways in which the examiner might help him or his family with their difficulties.

General Health (Psychophysiologic Status)

Psychophysiologic difficulties can be ascertained by inquiry into past sicknesses or injuries and the patient's reaction to these events. If she has not volunteered the information, she should be asked about current somatic symptoms; when appropriate, a menstrual history should be taken. Questions about eating habits, sleeping habits, and general physical well-being can be postulated. If one suspects poor contact with reality, inquiry can be made about any visions or voices.

On one occasion when the author was examining a 12-year-old boy who appeared to be responding to voices, inquiry was made about his general health and whether he had any hearing difficulties in the form of buzzing or sounds or speech that others did not seem to hear. The boy turned to the examiner and replied, "I beg your pardon, Doctor, but I do not have hallucinations."

The child may be asked to draw a person and then a person of the opposite sex and sign her name. If she will tell stories about the figures, these will increase the examiner's knowledge of the child's self-concept and interpersonal relations. At the very least, drawings will give some grasp of the child's fine motor coordination. The drawings may be used to score a rough estimate of the child's intelligence following the Goodenough Draw-a-Person Test.[6] Silver[8] has reviewed Goodenough's test and has added some ideas of his own on the diagnostic value of children's drawings of persons.

Fantasies and Fears

Much of the content of the interview may be the patient's fantasies. Any story he will tell or any game he will make up is part of his fantasy, as are his freehand drawings or paintings. No one fantasy is distinctively characteristic of any specific condition, but each can give impressions about the child's contact with reality, her intelligence, the predominant feelings she has, her concept of self, and her degree of inhibition or lack of inhibition as to feelings. If the child is willing to associate verbally and to display feelings in relation to fantasy productions, the unique meaning of the play can be revealed. Often play reflects family relationships or past experiences. Sometimes the child is so guarded and nonverbal we must enter into a "trial of treatment" based upon the history with relatively little first-hand knowledge of the child's thoughts and feelings. Alfred, age 7½, presented such a situation.

> Alfred was referred because of school failure, severe disability in reading, multiple somatic complaints, negativism with temper outbursts and night terrors. His parents had been divorced for approximately 14 months at the time of the referral. He and his two brothers lived in the custody of their mother. However, the matter of custody and particularly the father's visitation had remained an open battlefield. Although each parent seemed genuinely fond of the child and concerned about his symptoms, they blamed the other one for upsetting the boy and seemed to hope the psychiatric evaluation would recommend termination of visitation and the awarding of custody to him or her alone.
>
> During three diagnostic sessions, Alfred sat stiffly in a chair with his face turned to the wall, and he refused to talk to the examiner. It was impossible to establish eye contact or persuade him to play with any of the toys in the room. It was decided that we would have a trial of treatment, hoping that counseling of the parents would lessen the tension and that eventually the boy would interact with the therapist. Alfred continued the same behavior for two more sessions. Finally, on the sixth visit, after sitting for 15 or 20 minutes in his usual chair, Alfred did look around the room and went to the table to use the drawing materials. After a few minutes, the examiner walked over and sat down at the table to look over Alfred's shoulder. Alfred bent over and covered the drawing with his head and his hands, but continued to draw. He continued this activity for the remainder of the hour, and, when he was told our time was up, he took his papers, wadded them up into a ball and shoved them in his pocket.
>
> Over the next three visits, Alfred continued the drawing activities. Gradually, he would let the examiner see what he was doing, but he would not discuss his pictures and always took them with him. By the 10th interview, Alfred seemed much more relaxed and was sitting up straight so the examiner could get a full view of the things he was drawing. He was very meticulous and slow, bearing down heavily on the pencil, often breaking the lead. He drew two elaborate castles that had a medieval appearance. He added some figures in each turret. He

ran clotheslines from one turret to the other and hung wash on them. He then draw a tremendous number of arrows going back and forth from one turret to the other. The examiner asked him whether a war was going on, and he agreed that it was. The examiner commented that his mom and dad had a war going, too. At first, Alfred seemed startled and the therapist thought he had made a technical mistake that would possibly drive the child back to silence. However, after a few minutes, Alfred said he thought the examiner was right and talked about how much he hated his father. He was afraid his father would hurt his mother. Father was always screaming and yelling. Father was very preoccupied about health and supervised toothbrushing and diet very carefully. Candy was not permitted. He wished he didn't have to visit his father on weekends. It was scary and they never have any fun. Alfred thinks about his parents and the divorce all the time. He is scared in school because he thinks his father might come to kidnap him.

Over 9 or 10 months of individual psychotherapy accompanied by intensive counseling of the parents by another therapist, Alfred's temper outbursts, somatic complaints and nightmares gradually subsided. Academic performance improved with remedial reading, which was strongly resisted at first. With great difficulty, the parents ended their "war" and worked toward the spirit of joint custody. The parents took turns bringing Alfred to therapy, but the therapist maintained minimal contact with them in order to preserve his neutral status in the "war." Near the end of therapy Alfred was observed walking with his father, holding his hand and chatting amicably. T. commented that he and his father seemed to be friends again. Alfred replied, "Oh yes. Mrs. C. (father's therapist) has really helped him. He's a lot better."

Alfred was evaluated several years before DSM III was published. At that time we seldom used DSM II because it was not particularly useful and keeping statistics was not in vogue. Using DSM III we would classify him retrospectively as follows:

Axis I: Adjustment disorder with mixed disturbance of emotions and conduct plus academic inhibition

Axis II: Developmental reading disorder

Axis III: No physical illness

Axis IV: Stress: #5 Severe. Divorce of parents.

Axis V: Adaptive level past year #5. Poor. Doing poorly socially and academically. In 4th grade. Reading at grade 1.2 level and mathematics at grade 3.2 level.

It was our hope that most, if not all, of Alfred's problems were a direct reaction to the untoward parental situation, and deep refractory psychopathology had not yet occurred. In view of his superior intellectual abilities, his reading disability was a very serious problem. There was no family history of learning disabilities and no history of gestational or birth events suggesting central nervous system damage. However, he was observed to be somewhat clumsy and uncoordinated. Neuropsychologic testing showed a deficiency in visual form perception which could be interfering with the "development of appreciation of the symbolic and communicational significance of language and numerical symbols."

Two younger brothers did not seem especially upset by the divorce. It may have been because Alfred was the oldest or because of his learning disability that he became the focus of such intense parental conflict. No matter whether the cause of his reading disability was organic or functional his negativism and oppositional tendencies made the remedial program rather long and arduous, and it continued long after psychotherapy had ended. He was a sophomore in high school before he began doing his homework on his own. At the time of this writing he has completed one year of college; maintains a civil, but distant, relationship with his father, and has some concern over his lack of career choice. In a recent conversation he recalled the many sessions filled with stony silence. He chuckled and said he was so angry about being brought to see me that he vowed he would not talk. He cannot recall anything in particular that changed his mind. Although his grades have been satisfactory, he wishes he could read better. He also wishes he were closer to his father but believes the latter is such a difficult person that he (Alfred) must keep at a distance to avoid conflicts.

In addition to the child's spontaneous productions, one can inquire about his nicest dreams, his scariest dreams, and any repetitive dreams. One can ask for the earliest memory and for three wishes; these may often be associated with the deepest psychologic problems. One can offer the possibility of three money bags, with which the child may do anything, as a substitute for the question about three wishes.

Inquiry about fears and worries can be made directly from any clues the child may have given. Often the child feels that he is the only one with such fears or worries, and one may offer him reassurance. He can be asked his ideas about what happens to people who die and about any fears he may have about dying.

Some additional clues about the child's identification and her most problematic feelings can be learned by asking what kind of animal she would like to be and what particularly appeals to her about that animal.

Social Awareness

Often, by directly or indirectly inquiring about the limits of the playroom situation, the child reveals something of his concept of right and wrong or concern about possible loss of control. Occasionally the child may be asked directly whether he thinks certain acts are right or wrong and why he thinks so. Questions about social activities and interests will already have revealed a considerable amount about the social-cultural standards of the child's background. Matters of social control and limits, as well as a sense of right and wrong, may well be emotion-laden topics, the child already having had considerable experience with the differences between the adult's view and his own view of these matters. Hence any questions that must be asked should be framed in a nonjudgmental and fact-gathering manner. It is essential that the clinician also learn, directly or indirectly, the social attitudes of the child's family and community, to discover the degree of harmony or disharmony be-

tween the child and the parents and between the family and
their community.

SUMMARY

Interviewing techniques depend upon three variables: the
child, the examiner, and the examination setting. The setting
may be a playroom or office, but the author prefers a combination of both. Equipment should facilitate the child's verbal
and physical expressions. He may be taken out of the office or
building to facilitate the establishment of the relationship. In
the office there should be opportunities to talk or play. The
availability of a wide variety of toys and creative materials helps
the child freely express fantasies. Fantasies become clinically
meaningful to the examiner when the child verbalizes accompanying thoughts and the associated affect is noted.

Child psychiatrists need to recognize that their own emotions
are significant factors affecting both diagnostic and therapeutic
work. No absolute rule can be made about whether all child
psychiatrists should or should not have a personal psychoanalysis or psychotherapy as an essential part of training. Certainly a definite goal of the training should be the development
of insight into any aspect of the psychiatrist's personality that
may impair his effectiveness with patients. Whether analysis
or personal therapy is essential for the candidate's training is
a matter that he/she must decide for himself/herself in consultation with supervisors.

In general, children are highly resistive to psychiatric exploration and therapy. It is essential to recognize the reality basis
of much of the resistance. This is particularly true for delinquent children. Negativism and resistance to the psychiatrist's
efforts to relate to the child can be lessened somewhat by having
the utmost patience, using the open-end question whenever
possible, being open and aboveboard at all times, and making
every effort to avoid being or appearing judgmental.

Ten broad, general topics around which the author loosely
structures interviews have been listed. Considerable detail
about the child in each of these reference areas is needed. Examples of the kind and amount of detail needed are offered in
the discussion. It is hoped that the child will spontaneously
and freely reveal this information. When she/he does not, ex-

ploratory questions or activities that stimulate the child to reveal herself/himself should be used.

REFERENCES

1. Aichorn, A.: *Wayward Youth*. New York, Viking Press, 1925, 1935, 1965.
2. American Medical Association: Application for Certification in Child Psychiatry. *In* Directory of Residency Training Programs: accredited by the Accreditation Council for Graduate Medical Education. Chicago, A.M.A., 1985, pp. 528–530.
3. Beiser, H.R.: Psychiatric diagnostic interviews with children. J. Am. Acad. Child Psychiatry, *1*:656, 1962.
4. Erickson, E.H.: *Childhood and Society*. Rev. Ed. New York, W.W. Norton & Co., 1964, pp. 209–246.
5. Freud, A.: *Normality and Pathology in Childhood*. New York, International University Press, Inc., 1965, pp. 54–140.
6. Goodenough, F.L.: *Measurement of Intelligence by Drawings*. New York, World Book Co., 1926.
7. Martin, M.G.: Examination of the disturbed child. Curr. Med. Dig., *27*:57, 1960.
8. Silver, A.A.: Diagnostic value of three drawing tests for children. J. Pediatr., *37*:129, 1950.
9. Werkman, S.L.: The psychiatric diagnostic interview with children. Am. J. Orthopsychiatry, *35*:764, 1965.

4

THE MENTAL STATUS REPORT

Chapters 1 and 3 concentrated on techniques for interviewing children. This section will present an outline that we have found useful for organizing and recording the observations of the clinical interviews. Student physicians must learn to gather clinical data and write up the findings in a manner that is comprehensible and useful to them and their colleagues. The psychiatrist's account of first-hand observations of the patient constitutes the mental status report.

To facilitate professional communications and to increase objectivity and accuracy, it is essential to have a set of factors that can be regularly examined and systematically recorded for each child. Such factors must be items available for examination in a wide variety of children, definable with reasonable clarity, and capable of depicting qualitative and quantitative variations. In our practice we have used a modification of Beres's[1] systematic evaluation of ego functions of schizophrenic children. The observable aspects of the child's personality constitute his ego and the conscious part of his superego. These personality facets are present with variations in every child, whether severely disturbed or relatively healthy.

The categories presented here are not the only possible sub-headings that can be used for a mental status report. When properly defined, however, ego functions have provided us a good descriptive frame of reference. Terms such as *ego strength* and *ego adequacy* are not sufficient. The ego is not a thing but a group of related and overlapping functions. Freud[2] described the ego as a utilitarian part of the personality "entrusted with important functions." For our thesis it is not relevant to discuss the way that the ego functions develop. Rather, we intend to

list a group of psychic phenomena that, by common usage, have
come to be regarded as ego functions.

The mental status report is a description of the child's appearance and behavior during 2 or 3 hours of psychiatric interviews. If the ego functions outlined here are carefully examined, it is likely that neither significant pathology nor
personality strengths will be overlooked. The diagnosis can be
vague and confusing if important ego deviations are overlooked
and not recorded or if only deviant aspects of the personality
are noted, overlooking the more or less intact ego functions.

The listing of these items for the mental status report is not
intended as a regimentation of interviewing. It merely serves
as a standard guide for recording the kinds of observations
needed. Not all the items can be considered ego functions. Each,
however, either is an ego function or reflects upon one or more
ego functions. Ego functions do not separate distinctly, as the
movements of the right arm and of the left arm do. Therefore,
the division of these items has been rather arbitrary, as has the
order of their listing.

OUTLINE FOR MENTAL STATUS EXAMINATION
OF A CHILD

1. Appearance
2. Mood or affect
3. Orientation and perception
4. Coping mechanisms
   a. Major defenses
   b. Expression and control of affectional and aggres-
      sive impulses
5. Neuromuscular integration
6. Thought processes and verbalization
7. Fantasy
   a. Dreams
   b. Drawings
   c. Wishes
   d. Play
8. Superego
   a. Ego ideals and values
   b. Integration into personality
9. Concept of self
   a. Object relations

      b. Identifications
  10. Awareness of problems
  11. Intelligence quotient estimate
  12. Summary of mental status evaluation

Appearance

Appearance can give clues to ego functions, such as identifications that the child seems to be making, her need for conformity or nonconformity to various social groups, and her socioeconomic subculture. It is not enough to state that a child is dressed appropriately or inappropriately for her age and social group, since only your best friends will know what you mean and they may disagree with you. Some children are ardent conformists to nonconformist groups. Therefore, a description of the child's size, appearance, and manner of dress should be included as part of the mental status. Such characteristics as severe acne, obesity, and obvious handicaps should be noted as either possible causes or results of chronic emotional problems. Mannerisms, tics, and speech disturbances should always be recorded descriptively.

Mood or Affect

Mood or *affect* is the predominant feelings displayed by the patient. How does the mood fluctuate or change during the interview, from interview to interview or from topic to topic? Is the youngster able to demonstrate the full range of affect? For instance, a child may look flat or frightened in the beginning, but as he relaxes he may reveal that other feelings dominate his consciousness even more. The ease or lack of ease with which a child handles and displays different emotions is helpful in diagnostic assessments. Is the child particularly inhibited or uninhibited only in the first interview or throughout several diagnostic sessions? Brief observations of the patient in the waiting room may contrast with the child's playroom behavior and should be recorded.

Orientation and Perception

These ego functions reflect much about the child's ability to see and comprehend reality. In assessing the child's orientation, we are comparing her intellectual grasp of reality to her age and social peer group's knowledge of time, place, and person.

Perception refers to the kinds of impressions she gains about objects or events by the use of her special senses.

In assessing perception, we need to know to what extent she clearly differentiates fact from fantasy. By the age of 3 or 4 some ability to differentiate should be evident, and by 6 or 7 years a healthy child can make clear distinctions between her fantasy life and her reality situation.

In addition to clarifying which events are make-believe, we can ask him to tell about his clinic experience. If he was not told about the clinic, what kind of guesses does he make? Can he recount his trip to the clinic? Does he recognize the toys? Can he figure out the way to use a new toy he has never seen before? Does he respond to visual and auditory stimuli outside the room? How does he respond to the stimuli inside the room? Naturally, it is necessary to know that the perceptual mechanisms for sight, hearing, smell, touch, and so on, are organically intact.

Irrespective of the age of the child, it is important to observe which of the senses—sight, hearing, touch, and taste—are used. By noting the qualitative and quantitative use of these senses and using our clinical judgment, we can ascertain the age-appropriateness of the perceptive abilities. For example, it is age-appropriate for a 5-year-old to examine a variety of toys and objects in a room, using all the special senses, before selecting something that interests him. A 15-year-old would more appropriately explore the room with the eyes only and for a briefer time. Seriously disturbed children of any age vary from a constricted use of the sense organs to an extreme of hyperperceptiveness wherein minor stimuli appear to intrude themselves forcefully into consciousness.

Orientation is the patient's knowledge of objects and persons, including herself, and their relations in time and space. Does she know her name, address, birth date, seasons of the year, parents' occupation, and where she is? A true mental concept of time in terms of hours, weeks, and months is often not very clear to the child until about the age of 8 or 9. We need to know how far she has progressed in learning time relations and concepts. We can discern this by discussing events in her personal history and daily life and by noting the ability to understand time between clinic visits. When told that the next visit will be a week from today, at two o'clock, a 5- or 6-year-old may ask whether she will see you tomorrow, but such a question would be inappropriate for a 9- or 10-year-old.

Coping Mechanisms

Coping mechanisms are the ways in which the patient handles strong emotions, instinctual impulses, and nonspecific anxiety. What defense mechanisms does he try to use? Which defense mechanisms predominate in the interview? In other words, does he act out, deny, avoid, rationalize, intellectualize, project? Unfortunately, clinicians do not have absolute agreement on the precise definition of the defense mechanism terms. Even so, we must pay particular attention to the child's coping methods and mechanisms in our interviews. To avoid confusion, a verbal description of the child's behavior is recorded, omitting the use of psychologic jargon or reserving such terms to brief conclusions in the summary. The following example illustrates this.

> The body of a mental status report contained a direct observation in which Harold, age 11 years, claimed he knew all about babies. When pressed to tell what he knew he seemed startled and confused but then quickly replied: "Oh, yes, that's the one where your father starts out, 'Now, son, I've noticed you're at the age when you should know certain things'—I know all about babies. I don't want to talk about that stuff any more."
>
> Referring to this observation, the summary of the report contained the following: "Discussion of sexual matters provoked anxiety in Harold that he tried to handle intellectually but then could only handle by evading and avoiding the subject."

Intellectualization, evasion, and avoidance are healthy defense mechanisms if not used excessively. The actual clinical significance of this boy's reactions can be assessed only in relation to the total case work-up and cannot be considered *a priori* evidence of a serious sexual problem. The introduction of the topic of sex did produce obvious anxiety, as it does in most children of this age.

The point to be made here is that accurately recorded mental status examinations can be used to assess changes in the patient that occur over periods of time. If only the summary had been recorded, it would have been impossible to assess qualitative changes in the child's knowledge and reactions about sex unless all subsequent examinations were made by the original examiner who had an infallible memory.

Diversions of the course of play or conversation constitute a

form of coping used by patients of all ages. When this phenomenon occurs, the examiner may assume that the child is trying
consciously or unconsciously to cope with anxiety. Is the source
of the anxiety the situation of coming to the physician, something about the physician himself, the subject matter of the play,
or a high degree of anxiety related to deeper problems that
plague the child regardless of the subject or setting?

Space will not permit a comprehensive list of the innumer-
able varieties of coping mechanisms used by individual children. I assume that every person has affectional and aggressive
impulses that must be handled at the ego level. Everyone also
has anxiety from a variety of other sources and functions in
certain ways that he has learned to keep the anxiety at the lowest
possible level for him. I am therefore interested in how successful his coping mechanisms are (1) in relieving feelings of
anxiety and (2) in facilitating individual functioning. Note the
contrast in the following two cases:

> *Case 1.* Betsy, age 7½, silently took the examiner's hand and went to
> the playroom. She did not speak or look at the examiner. Her facial
> expression was blank. After only a momentary glance around the room
> she crawled under the play table, pulled her knees up to her chest, and
> closed her eyes. She did not move when the examiner touched her. Her
> pulse and breathing were slow and steady.
>
> *Case 2.* Billy, age 8, appeared inordinately frightened but would look
> at the examiner and whisper brief answers to questions. The examiner
> tried to talk to him about the scary feelings children often have when
> they go to the doctor. He said that this was all news to him and that he
> had never had any of those feelings. His pupils were widely dilated, and
> his breathing was rapid. Since talking did not make him feel relieved,
> the examiner invited him to use the playroom facilities and materials.
> Billy merely sat and squirmed in the chair. The examiner's silence
> seemed to make him even more anxious. The examiner then took the
> initiative to divert him into a game. Billy complied with instructions
> but never relaxed. When the time was up, he could not get down the
> hall fast enough. None of the mechanisms he used and none of the
> technics the examiner used had been completely successful in relieving
> the anxiety.

One may spectulate that Betsy was overwhelmed by anxiety.
On the other hand, one could also speculate that she was free
of conscious anxiety since she did not show any of its usual
physical concomitants. Even if we conclude that her withdrawal successfully relieved her of a conscious feeling of anxiety, we must also conclude that her methods of coping with
the situation were such that her total functioning was seriously
impaired.

Billy showed a high degree of anxiety, which he was unable

to relieve and which affected his ability to relate to the examiner and to use the toy room for his own pleasure. His anxiety was greatly relieved by the termination of the interview, but he did not totally withdraw from the examiner until given permission to do so.

The behavior of both children was so significantly different from that of the average child that we felt safe in concluding that their reactions were not solely in response to the immediate environment. Although both children used avoidance and withdrawal, Billy's behavior more nearly approximated the psychosocial behavior of his age group. Additional interviews with both children, spaced at intervals of several days or a week, were indicated to explore other areas of their functioning and to learn whether familiarity with the examiner and the surroundings would lessen the anxiety response to the clinic visits themselves.

Billy's behavior changed only slightly in two subsequent diagnostic interviews. On the basis of history and other findings, it was concluded that he was suffering a severe neurotic adjustment reaction brought on by an extremely traumatic home situation, and a trial of weekly therapy sessions with him and his parents on an outpatient basis was instituted. As he relaxed during the ensuing weeks and months, the physical signs of anxiety disappeared. He became able to use the toys in structured games and finally became able to indulge in fantasy play and conversation with the therapist.

Betsy's behavior had been essentially as described for several months. She was hospitalized for further study. It seemed that some of her sleepiness might have been an untoward response to previous tranquilizing medication. Discontinuation of all medication did result in a wider variety of behavior, but communication with others by touch, gesture, or eye contact remained minimal, and she never spoke more than a few unintelligible words in a singsong manner. Although both of these children could be said to be manifesting avoidance and denial, on qualitative assessment Betsy is by far the sicker of the two.

Neuromuscular Integration

We need to know the degree of activity of the child and to observe gross and fine movements. How does she handle a ball? Can she handle the mechanical toys? Are movements smooth or jerky? Very young children, some psychotic children, some infantilized children, and some brain-damaged children show varying degrees of difficulty with motility and coordination.

Thought Processes and Verbalization

Information about the child's spontaneous speech and verbalization is often available as soon as you meet him. I also include his play as part of spontaneous thinking.

> Dr. Z reported a "frustrating" interview with Christopher. "I didn't learn a thing because he just wouldn't talk to me." The supervisor asked what the child had done. "Well, he just sat there and drew. He wouldn't look at me or talk to me. He drew a house, and then there were some figures put on the house, and then he wouldn't discuss the drawing. Then he scribbled over it with black crayon."

Chris' home situation had an abundance of severe problems. Even though silent with the examiner, he failed to hide the fact he was preoccupied with a home and the people in it. Play is thinking, albeit partly unconscious. We cannot be absolutely certain of the personal psychological meaning of a drawing unless the child is willing to talk about it. The point here is that the examiner need not have been so "frustrated." When children draw they are trying to tell something. In reviewing this interview, I felt that Chris wanted to talk about his home but was afraid to reveal the details just yet.

I am interested in the rate, sequence, form, and quality of the thinking and in any special preoccupations the child has. Often in spontaneous play or conversations certain themes recur that give clues to problem areas. As clinicians we are interested in problems and the child's views of his symptoms. Yet, as noted in a previous section, children seldom, if ever, have a part in the decision to seek help, and it is not surprising that most children cannot or will not discuss "problems." Indeed, we always consider ourselves fortunate if a child will engage in spontaneous conversation about any topic of interest to him. Just letting him talk provides much information about his vocabulary, his sociocultural milieu, his interests, his relationships, his ability to relate, and his ability to organize his thinking.

Fantasy

In the outline at the beginning of this chapter, we included dreams, drawings, wishes, and much of the play activity as subdivisions of fantasy. Fantasy is a part of the thinking processes. It is also a reflection of other ego functions. Sometimes fantasy is used as a major coping mechanism. The child's fantasies also can reveal much about her perceptive and intellectual abilities. Fantasy play or stories usually reveal problematic areas in the child's intrapsychic and interpersonal experiences. Quantitative and qualitative aspects of fantasy production are important diagnostically. Yet neither fantasy nor any other single part of the mental status evaluation can be considered conclusive or pathognomonic of any specific condition.

From clinical experience we know that the severely hedonistic, relaxed, glib, acting-out child usually displays a dearth of fantasy material. These children do not remember or are unwilling to tell about dreams. Their wishes either are for concrete, material objects of great value or are exaggeratedly altruistic. "I can't think of three wishes. The only one is that there never be any more wars and everyone everywhere will always be happy" was the pious wish expressed by one 11-year-old whose history was replete with antisocial acting-out behavior. He engaged in no fantasy play and was evasive and brief when the examiner attempted to engage him in storytelling. Although his wish seemed to be presented as a conscious effort to tell the examiner what a nice, good boy he is, it also implied a wish to alter or abolish the violent aggression and resultant unhappiness in himself and his world.

There may also be a low quantity of fantasy material in highly anxious, extremely inhibited, neurotic or schizoid children. In these cases the verbal inhibitions are not so selective as with the acting-out child. At the opposite extreme, some acutely psychotic children may show that fantasy dominates most of their waking hours, nearly excluding reality considerations.

Qualitatively, fantasies that deal with real life problems indicate a reasonably healthy use of fantasy as a coping device in both healthy and moderately neurotic children. Such phenomena are seen in children who use doll play to act out, perhaps ventilate, their experiences of visits to the physician or the dentist, a hospitalization, or the loss of a loved pet or playmate. Fantasies replete with sadism, sexually symbolic behavior, and megalomanic world destruction, with little or no relevance to the child's reality situation, are seen in borderline psychotic and severely neurotic children. Overtly schizophrenic adolescents who permit adults to learn their fantasies are likely to reveal undifferentiated sexual-aggressive ideas of bizarre content with tangential and dissociated themes. The impression is a flood of confused, garbled thoughts.

Whether the fantasies are revealed through free play, drawing, dreams, or wishes, it is always important for the examiner to assess the child's ability to distinguish fantasy from reality. Students frequently complain that supervisors stretch their imaginations to make something significant out of the child's play. After all, dreams are dreams and play is play. Students often ask, "Since all children indulge in fantasy, how can you tell normal from abnormal fantasies?"

The question discloses the medical students' wish to oversimplify diagnosis by easily and sharply separating normal and pathologic phenomena. Except for extremely bizarre, violent, or overtly sexual fantasy play or verbalizations, the content often does not reveal either pathology or normalcy. It is usually not possible to answer the question of "How pathologic?" on the basis of content alone. We are interested in whether a child uses fantasy in a healthy or unhealthy way and whether he can distinguish it from reality. More importantly, we want to know the child's thoughts and feelings. Fantasy permits a child to reveal his thoughts and feelings to an adult more comfortably than does direct conversation. He may not know that he is talking about himself as he makes up play or tells a story. Should he suddenly realize that he is revealing intimate thoughts, or should his thoughts frighten him, he can always relieve the attending anxiety by reminding the examiner that it is all "make-believe."

It is common practice to ask for the child's three wishes. Sometimes they wish for something that will obviously change a problematic situation, such as "I wish my mother and daddy wouldn't be divorced any more." Often the child's wishes are merely popular, common ones. Like the popular Rorschach responses, they do not give clues to problem areas. Common wishes do indicate, however, that some of the child's thinking is in tune with that of his peer group. "Affectionless" and dependency-deprived children do not talk about needing love and security. They are likely to wish for food, money, or lavish material possessions. Often inquiry into what a child would do if the wish were granted produces clarifying fantasies.

Much of the same can be said about dreams. Many children enjoy telling their scariest, nicest, most recent, or repetitive dreams. Children cannot free-associate to their dreams, and this is probably not desirable, since the examiner always treads a narrow path between learning as much as he can and yet avoiding the stimulation of overwhelming anxiety. Nevertheless, the more details a child gives about his dreams, the more one learns about the thoughts he has when the conscious censor or guard is asleep at the gate. Sometimes repetitive dreams of violence or dreams with thinly disguised sexual themes give the only clue to the source of conflict in an anxious but otherwise well-adjusted child. Dreams are particularly useful in helping us understand some adolescents.

It goes almost without saying that free play not only helps put the child at ease with the adult examiner but also reveals emotional expressions and thoughts about herself and the world around her. Drawings and the child's discussions of such productions are useful in the same ways. For the use of drawings in a more standardized manner as diagnostic aids the reader is referred to the works of Goodenough[3] and Silver.[4]

Much more research needs to be done if drawings or spontaneous fantasies of any form are to become standardized projective techniques. Children's free play and fantasies offer such a rich source of information about them as individuals on an empirical basis alone that one questions whether further standardization of this material is necessary, desirable, or even possible.

Superego

We can observe or examine only the conscious part of the superego. We are interested in the child's ideals and value system. To what extent does his concept of good and bad or right and wrong seem to influence his behavior? Does he seem preoccupied with antisocial or forbidden impulses? If so, is the result of excessive constriction of behavior or an opposite lack of control? When there is lack of control, either the impulse to act out is inordinately strong or the child is totally dependent upon the external environment to set limits because internalization has not occurred. Sometimes these children have identified with antisocial adults and have internalized a corrupt superego. The constricted child may also suffer pressure from strong impulses to act out. Such children have either incorporated a rigid superego or the fear of loss of control and inability to judge acceptable limits make "no action" the only possible mode of behavior. Little boys who have been labeled a "sissy" or "coward" by peers should always be asked their thoughts and feelings during a confrontation or fight. Many deny having fear of bodily harm but can recall feelings of terror and dismay over a brief conscious awareness of their own homicidal potential.

Naturally, it is important to know their intellectual concepts of right and wrong. Beyond that, we should try to learn the discrepancies between stated standards and actual, internalized standards. Is the superego a source of frequent or constant anxiety, or is it an automatic regulator of behavior that helps avoid anxiety-producing situations and thus actually facilitates social interactions? Children with serious superego conflicts may deny even the mildest aggressive or sexual impulses. They are often oversolicitous of others (reaction formation), guilt-ridden, or compulsive; have a poor self-concept, and are prone to somatic symptoms.

Concept of Self

We put concept of self, object relations, and identification in a group together because these aspects of the ego seem intimately related and do not permit a separate discussion or examination. It seems to be splitting hairs to try to make distinct categories out of each of these. For instance, the child's concept of himself is closely tied to his identifications and to the kinds of relations he has established with other people.

Beres[1] states that the child develops from narcissism to true object relations, from inadequate self-awareness to self-identity, from transient identifications to the permanent identifications that lead to ego and superego formation. The immature human being goes from confusion of identity to a definitive sexual identity. The development of all these aspects is in active, dynamic flux in the child, subject to progression and regression according to the various inner and outer forces acting on her at any given time. Diagnostically, we are interested in the qualitative and quantitative aspects of the self-concept, the object relations, and the identifications as the child reveals them at the time of the examination. The central issue of determining whether there is retardation of development or regression from a more developed state must rely on accurate history and often on prolonged observation for an answer.

Does the child see herself as strong or weak, good or bad, large or small, pretty or ugly, and in comparison with whom? How does she approach and interact with the examiner? From direct observation, from the play, and from the conversation, how would one describe the feelings that predominate in her daily negotiations with parents and siblings? What are the number and the depth of her friendships? How does she characterize the people in the world? The child's self-concept can be graphically portrayed with the following game.

SELF-RATING CHART
(How do you see yourself?)

Compare yourself with others: 10 is the highest score and 1 is lowest. Put an X in the square where you belong. Use the red pencil when comparing yourself with classmates at school. Use the green pencil when comparing yourself with people in your family.

	Handsomest (Prettiest)	Tallest	Strongest	Smartest	Best Liked	
10						10
9						9
8						8
7						7
6						6
5						5
4						4
3						3
2						2
1						1
	Ugliest	Shortest	Weakest	Dumbest	Hated	

The examiner should do this exercise with the patient to make it more fun and to be certain the patient understands that it is his/her opinion we want. Many children tend to underrate themselves, out of a sense of modesty. However, some forthrightly rate themselves quite accurately. Still others are grossly inaccurate, especially in the columns relating to intelligence and physical strength. The "Best Liked" column is usually the child's honest appraisal of the way he believes others feel about him.

The last three items on the list—awareness of problems, intelligence quotient estimate, and summary of the mental status evaluation—are not ego functions. They do not need special definition and will not be discussed further.

SUMMARY

The child psychiatrist must be able to comprehend his patients as distinct, functioning individuals. His comprehension of the patient is tested by his ability to write the findings and clearly communicate them to colleagues. I have offered a list of ego functions as a moderately standardized frame of reference for describing children as they are seen during examination. It is my thesis that diagnosis is improved if the physician concentrates on describing both the assets and the liabilities of the personality. We must control our urges to delineate sharply the "pathologic" from the "normal" until we understand the person and have at least a historical overview of his life situation.

My experience has been that the use of this list of ego functions as a mental status examination outline promotes depth and thoroughness of examination by our student psychiatrists. It has the additional advantage of providing a graphic account of the child that can be used for comparison later.

The mental status report is a cross-sectional word picture of the child at a given time, under special circumstances. The clinical significance of these findings increase in value as they are related to the child's sociofamilial situation and past history. The outline for case study and the case summaries in subsequent chapters illustrate the integration of the mental status report with other clinical data.

REFERENCES

1. Beres, D.: Ego deviations and the concept of schizophrenia. In *The Psychoanalytic Study of the Child.* Vol. 11. New York, International Universities Press, Inc., 1956, p. 164.
2. Freud, S.: *The Ego and the Id.* London, Hogarth Press, 1927, 1950, pp. 81–88.
3. Goodenough, F.L.: *Measurement of Intelligence by Drawings.* New York, World Book Co., 1926.
4. Silver, A.A.: Diagnostic value of three drawing tests for children. J. Pediatr., *37*:129, 1950.

5

MENTAL STATUS PROFILES: NORMAL AND ABNORMAL

The emphasis of this text has been upon the diagnostic assessment of children rather than on a review of the established and theoretical knowledge about various nosological categories. The reader should keep in mind that appraisal of the ego functions of a specific child is useful only in estimating the severity of the illness. Such appraisals cannot be used as a basis for diagnostic classification, since classification includes etiologic and prognostic considerations that are not evident from the mental status examination alone.

Unfortunately, it is easier to measure degrees of dysfunction than relative states of health. It would be impossible and presumptuous to attempt to draw a "normal" mental status profile for every age level. However, a discussion of the extremes of distortion seen in clinical practice and the range of normal variability for the ego functions listed in the preceding chapter seems feasible. Some generalizations about age-appropriateness of behavior, the significance of quantitative aberrations, and various combinations of ego deficits are also possible.

THREE PRESCHOOL BOYS

Each of the following three preschool youngsters behaved differently on examination. The fact that each of them was referred because of "suspected infantile autism" is illustrative of the confusion that has arisen over the term *autism,* even in sophisticated circles. The reader is asked to compare these children not only in terms of their total behavior but in terms of which ego functions were impaired and the extent of their impairment.

Mental Status Examinations

Case 1. Pete, age 2½ years: Peter was met in the waiting room. He smiled and went eagerly to the playroom, taking my hand. He talked spontaneously in complete sentences and could be well understood. He expressed an interest in the water and then went about the room examining the toys, settling for a baby doll. He asked me to put a bib on the doll and fix a bottle for her. He then fed her. After a period of this he went to the dollhouse, took out the furniture, and placed it on a play table. He identified the various pieces of furniture and commented about some of the broken ones' being unusable. He complained of the refrigerator's being broken, too, but accepted the explanation that it was just a toy, not designed to be opened. After some 10 minutes of doll play, he went to the sandbox and took a car out of it. He then reached and complained that he couldn't get a plane out. This was obtained for him, and he complained that he couldn't get another plane. He was asked whether he wanted to get in the sandbox, and he said he did. Permission was given and he climbed into the sandbox, climbing in and out many times, playing enthusiastically with the planes and with the sand. He would make the planes fly and land with appropriate noises and sometimes would stop and spontaneously identify the various parts of the plane. After a period of sand play he went about the room, enthusiastically examining the many other toys he found. He asked for some clay and played with it for a while, explaining, "You don't eat this." He then returned to the baby and bottle, playing with them for a while.

I asked Pete to draw for me, and he was very resistive to this, wanting to go back to his own play. However, he did cooperate after a few minutes and was able to copy a line and a circle, but he complained that he couldn't copy a box and he refused to try to draw a figure.

He was observed in some spontaneous play with his 4-year-old sister for a few minutes. They played quite easily together for a short time and then began to fight over the toys. It was noticed that Pete held his own and the sister began to cry. The mother came up and complained that they were embarrassing her. She separated them and said that she would take care of them when she got home.

Case 2. Billy, age 2 years, 5 months: Billy is an attractive child, appearing sturdy and well built with good muscular coordination. Alone with me in the examination room he was extremely upset at being separated from his mother. Because I could not console him, I asked the mother to join me in the examination. He sat on her lap, or extremely close to her feet when he was on the floor. As soon as he was comfortable and sure that I was not going to separate him from his mother again, he became interested in the toys. He played with a total of seven different toys, using all of them appropriately. He pushed the lawnmower back and forth on the floor. He played the musical book briefly. He asked his mother to read from the animal noise book and pulled the strings to make the animal sounds after his mother showed him how to do it. He took the top off the Tinker Toys and put a stick in a wheel. He tried to spin a top, unsuccessfully, because the top was broken. He pushed the train briefly and played with the wind-up bear three different times. He perceived the winding mechanism, tried to wind it unsuccessfully, then handed the toy to me to get it working. In the drawing maneuver, he sat on his mother's lap, picked up a crayon spontaneously, drew a straight line after demonstration, and scribbled after I demonstrated a circle. He used a circular motion after I demonstrated it but was never able to draw just individual circles.

I frustrated Billy by taking candy away from him. He was able to use a socially appropriate method of getting the candy from me by asking me please to give him the candy.

Case 3. Steven, age 3 years, 4 months: Steven is a chunky, willful child of enormous strength who can go quickly from one emotion to another. He could fly into an angry withdrawal, only to smile happily the next moment. He was the same with his mother. When he kicked at her, she told him to stop and held his legs firmly. The she smiled and tickled him, and he responded with a giggle. Once he retreated under the couch during the neurologic examination, and she lured him out merely by rolling the toy sweeper beside him. If he wanted something, he could generally be distracted by some other object.

His approach to me was sometimes babyish and sometimes bizarre. On first coming to my office, he reacted with fear to the movie camera and took refuge behind my chair. When I turned my head toward him and said something reassuring, he put his fingers on my eyelids, an action he often does at home with his parents and his dog.

Steven's response to adaptive tasks was as follows:

1. Ball play—he refused, although he picked up the ball after a pointing cue.
2. Ring stack set—he took rings off the stick but gave no indication that he understood the names of sizes or colors; his repositioning the rings was done well with some attention to size, and he made several corrections showing some appreciation of the nature of the apparatus. His final position of the rings was not correct.
3. Cowboy and Indian—of the materials offered he accepted with alacrity the horses and cows, lining them in a row. He seemed generally oblivious to my attempts to play but let me parallel play and looked at me.
4. Candy—he opened the opaque box immediately but needed to have the top pulled off the transparent one. He at first played with the M & M's, then ate them after I put one in his mouth. He ignored the wrapped candy. His coordination was adequate.
5. Drawing—he drew a straight line after demonstration. To other requests, he made a controlled scribble. He held his crayon in his fist.

His verbal behavior consisted of imitating a train and babbling. He made little effort to communicate with me, although he was not a difficult child to "read." Mostly he wanted to do what he wanted when he wanted, but he could be led, with some resistance, to try a new task if too much was not demanded. He understood some of what I said. I asked him where his mama was. An anxious expression came to his face. He got off my lap, took my hand, and led me to the door. He seemed to use my physical presence for comfort when he sought it but did not allow me much latitude in my approach to him, preferring to structure the interaction in a strict way.*

Comparison of the Mental Status of These Three Boys

The reader who has had no experience observing preschool children in a nonclinical setting is urged to arrange some ob-

---

*I am indebted to Dr. Marian K. DeMyer for the case material of Bill and Steven.

servation periods as a part of training. Only through actually watching children of this age group can one develop an appreciation for the wide range of normal behavior and at the same time sense the extremes that are beyond the range of normality. Those experienced with preschoolers will immediately be aware that the mental status examination of Pete, the first child, failed to reveal any striking abnormalities. Steven, the third patient, showed marked abnormal behavior in most areas, and Billy's overall functioning fell somewhere between that of Pete and Steven. The referral complaints for these boys mentioned periods of severe withdrawal interspersed with episodic emotional outbursts, various misbehaviors, and sleep pattern disruptions. The possibility of "infantile autism" was included in the differential considerations of each of the referring persons. A comparison of the ego functions, as outlined in Chapter 4, for each of these children explicitly differentiates them from one another.

APPEARANCE. The boys do not differ in that each had good physical development and was free of any stigmata or mannerisms.

MOOD OR AFFECT. In this area the differences are quite striking. None of the boys showed obvious sadness, which is an affective expression difficult to differentiate from frustration and anger in a very small child. They all revealed a full range of emotion, from happiness to fear to rage. For Pete the prevailing mood appears to have been contentment in happy—at times exuberent—play, whereas a tense fearfulness pervaded Billy's interview. Considering his age and the circumstances, Billy's inability to separate from mother is not considered so unusual. However, the panic-like clinging to the mother persisted during the next five interviews. Steven's moods were so variable and wide-range that one is at a loss to assign a "prevailing" mood to the interview hour. Pete illustrated a smooth, modulated transition from one affect to another, with the changes' being readily comprehensible in terms of the immediate environment. By contrast, the other boys' emotional expressions were sudden, unpredictable, and more intense. Billy's emotionality was easily modulated by the presence of the mother, whereas Steven's emotional outbursts were extremely difficult to change.

COPING MECHANISMS. The boys' methods of handling their feelings, anxieties, and frustrations were immature and numerically few because all of them actually are chronologically immature.

In addition to direct expression of angry impulses, all three used or attempted to use evasion, avoidance, and withdrawal to the point of appearing obstinate. However, Billy did this much less when his mother was present, and Pete defied the examiner only once, when the request for figure drawings was beyond his abilities. All of the patients tried to manipulate the environment, but again Pete was by far the most sophisticated. He made direct verbal requests for the examiner's participation and once by strong hints obtained permission to climb into the sandbox. Pete demonstrated awareness of adult restrictions and controlled an impulse to eat clay by offering an adult quotation, "You don't eat this." Neither of the other boys demonstrated this much ability to use the adult for either personal gratification or control of unacceptable wishes.

PERCEPTION AND ORIENTATION. Each of the boys appeared to be oriented correctly to his own name and to his mother. We do not expect precise orientation to time and place at this age, and these items were not checked. Perceptual ability is also limited at this age: at least, the child's limited language makes it impossible for him to tell us his understanding of the objects and events in his environment. By inference from the children's play it appeared that Steven had the least ability to differentiate the toys by size, color, or appropriate use. It is impossible to tell whether this apparent perceptual deficit was due to poor comprehension, inattention, or lack of motivation to perform.

THOUGHT PROCESSES AND VERBALIZATIONS. Without fairly extensive conversation, it is impossible to ascertain the thinking of another human being. However, when a child is engaged in some activity we can reasonably assume his thought processes are active. Steven's behavior was so unusual and unpredictable that it seems very likely that his thinking was quite unconventional. His verbal ability was similar to that seen in children 8 to 12 months of age. Billy had language ability, but fear and poor motivation reduced his productivity so that the actual vocabulary level remained uncertain.

FANTASY. For preschool children, fantasy play with a paucity of verbal accompaniment is usual. Therefore, attempts to describe these children's fantasies separately from coping or thinking behavior would be redundant. Fantasy content can only be accurately obtained from what the child will or can tell you about his play and dreams.

SUPEREGO. Internalization of the superego is still developing in the 2- to 4-year-old. As was mentioned, only Pete gave clear evidence of being aware of adult "do's and don'ts."

CONCEPT OF SELF AND OBJECT RELATIONS. These boys clearly illustrated different ways of relating to the examiner and to their mothers. Relations with peers and other adults were not observed and can only be surmised. All of them made eye contact and permitted touching. Steven's act of putting his finger on the eyelids of the examiner, his parents, and his dog is behavior that is seen infrequently and usually disappears well before 12 months of age. Steven showed relatively little differentiation between his mother and the examiner in his behavior reactions until the examiner specifically mentioned the mother. Billy sharply differentiated between the mother and the examiner and clung to his mother in fear. Such behavior is found commonly at 8 to 10 months, but persistence with such intensity (five interviews) to age 2½ is quite inappropriate. By contrast, the examiner remarked about Pete, "It was fun to be with him." Psychosexual identifications are hardly measurable at such a young age. It should be noted, however, that Pete's doll-baby play is not unusual for a 2½-year-old boy and modern parents now encourage doll play for little boys.

Relation of Mental Status to the Final Diagnosis

To the reasonably sophisticated reader it may seem surprising that all three of these very different little boys, ages 40 months, 29 months and 30 months of age, were referred because of "suspected infantile autism." Perhaps the referring person completely lacked knowledge or carelessly used the terms. It is more than 40 years since Leo Kanner[2] described a symptom complex that he named *infantile autism*. Much attention has been given this phenomenon in the hopes of making early diagnoses and finding effective treatments. Most medical students, if exposed to mental disorders of preschool children at all, have been taught to "rule out" mental retardation and childhood psychosis (infantile autism), which carry a uniformly bad prognosis. Less obvious developmental problems in preschool children probably are not covered in the medical school curriculum, especially when they occur in children who are free of any diagnosable physical or neurologic problem. With this educational background, most physicians either do not recognize emotional or mental disorders in preschool children or feel limited to three diagnostic possibilities, namely, mental retardation, autism or normal. The presenting complaints for each of these boys were periods of withdrawal interspersed with explosive outbursts and little or no "normal" response to discipline. With this history, none of them could be called normal. There were no conspicuous signs of mental retardation, an often extremely difficult diagnosis to make prior to age 5 or 6. Withdrawal, emotionality and negativism do occur in infantile autism. A presumptive diagnosis of autism, therefore, had some fallacious logic.

The 1980 *DSM III*[1] lists eight classes of mental disturbances in addition to retardation and autism that can and do appear in the preschool child. Autism is classified as one of the Pervasive Developmental Disorders. These disorders are characterized by actual distortions, not just delays, in such basic psychological functions as attention, perception, reality testing and motor movement, leading to serious problems in the development of social skills and language.

An accurate diagnosis can never be made on the mental status examination alone, no matter how prolonged or thoroughly performed. A complete present, past and family history along with the physical exam are also essential ingredients of the diagnostic work-up. Sometimes prolonged observation, even a trial of treatment, is needed for diagnosis. However, the mental status can help differentiate among the 45 possible diagnoses listed in *DSM III* by pointing toward certain possible conditions and away from others.

Of the three boys described, only Steven showed distortions in his behavior of sufficient degree that Autism had to be given serious consideration. However, many of his symptoms are also seen in children with mild mental retardation, Attention Deficit Disorder, Early Conduct Disorder or Oppositional Disorder. After additional observations, personal and family histories, intellectual (developmental) testing and a trial of treatment over several months, it was concluded that Steven indeed suffered a Pervasive Developmental Disorder. The onset had really been apparent at about 18 to 24 months of age. Although he did not have complete inability to respond to other people (review behavior with mother and examiner), he showed sufficient symptoms and behavioral distortions to justify the diagnosis of Pervasive Developmental Disorder, Autism.

Peter did not show either developmental delays or distortions in two sessions in addition to the reported one. He did not display the withdrawal, temper outbursts or negativism described by his parents. Attention span, reality awareness, language, social and motor skills were all age-appropriate. Birth, milestones and physical state were all normal. With some probing, it was learned the parents' marriage was in a very serious state of stress. The mother had denied marital problems to her family physician out of embarrassment and with the hope that Pete could be helped without getting into his parents' "mess." Mother was depressed and lonely. Father was "away" most of the time. Parental arguments were frequent. Pete's "periods of withdrawal" had not been observed by people other than the mother. However, when he was quietly by himself she believed he might be as sad and miserable as she. He did have tantrums (2½-year-old). Mother couldn't handle these and usually gave in to him. Father would spank him in anger, which would upset mother very much. His 2-year-old negativism distressed both parents. The parents' were told that their problems have the potential of affecting Pete's development adversely. With the usual delays and resistances these parents did accept a referral for marriage counseling. It was recommended that Peter begin having some nursery school experience 2 or 3 half-days per week to help his social skills and that he return to the psychiatric clinic every 4 months for a "check-up". We lost track of this family after 1½ years. When Pete was last seen shortly after his fourth birthday his development socially and emotionally was quite satisfactory. The parents were still living together and still in marriage therapy.

Our record of long-term follow-up for "at risk" children is rather poor and for that we are sorry. Many such "at risk" children seem to do rather well but many suffer a great deal and we can't help them if we don't see them and their families over long periods of time. In the case of Billy, his negativism was not intense, or, at least, seemed to be of the amount usually seen in the 2- to 3-year-old. His language and motor skills were also age-appropriate. His separation anxiety and withdrawal behavior were excessive, in degree, even for a much younger child, and gave a picture of overanxiety. In spite of poor social skills, no actual distortions of the development were found. There were many serious family problems that could be interfering with the development. Mother was overtly anxious and overprotective. Parents were divorced and relations with maternal grandmother were tumultuous. Father and maternal uncle both suffered from psychosis. On direct examination, Billy was not seen to be suffering autism. By both history and direct observation, Billy was seen as suffering an Overanxious Disorder as well as being at risk for further developmental and emotional disturbances.

Billy and his mother were referred to the mental health clinic in their hometown for outpatient treatment. The referral was accepted and they did attend the clinic, but the final outcome is not known. The chronically high anxiety level in the child and mother, the family history of psychosis, the severity and chronicity of the stress and the multiple family problems made the long-term prognosis rather guarded.

TWO SCHOOL-AGE GIRLS

The school initiated the referrals of the two 8-year-old girls whose mental status examinations are reported next. Neither child was making satisfactory academic progress in spite of high average (Abby) and superior intelligence (Jane). The school complained that Abby was so boisterous and destructive in the classroom that she could no longer be contained there. Jane's behavior was exemplary, but she did not seem "to grasp the academic material or know the answers." The school had recommended repeating the third grade for Jane and had requested that Abby be withdrawn from school after her failure to improve in a special class for emotionally disturbed children.

Mental Status Examinations

Case 1. Jane, age 8 years, 5 months: Jane had no physical abnormalities. She was neatly dressed and groomed for an 8-year-old. During the family intake conference, Jane sat quietly and did not attempt to speak even when spoken to. She hesitated briefly when asked to come for an individual interview. She entered the play therapy room and stood rooted by the door. She did not turn her head to explore the room visually but only looked at me, occasionally giving a furtive side glance about the room. She refused to sit or explore the room even when invited. She did not speak but only grimaced painfully and wrung her hands fretfully. She would not participate in any games with me and would not move from her fixed position. When I left the room she explored it quickly, painting a female figure and then drawing an excellent reproduction of a horse on the blackboard. She then returned to her original spot and stood there until I reentered the room. I then attempted to interest her in the dollhouse, but she refused to talk or move. When I again left the room she rearranged the doll house and resumed her former position before I returned. She eagerly joined her parents at the session's close.

At the second interview 1 week later, Jane again appeared quite anxious. However, she sat down when invited and talked much more freely. She still wrung her hands and grimaced during the conversation. She enunciated well, but there were occasional gaps in her knowledge. For instance, she did not know when her birthday was but only that it was during school and before the rest of the family's. In comparing Indianapolis and her hometown she could only say that there were more hospitals and taller buildings in Indianapolis. Jane stated that she reads during gym class because she doesn't like to play. She made good grades but her teacher thought she needed help with reading and sounding. She mentioned two bad boys in her room. When asked why they were bad she replied that one makes low marks and the other talks, so they get whipped. She then denied ever being whipped. She related several fears consisting of the following: she's afraid to sleep alone because the trees make shadows on the walls, and she's afraid people look in her upstairs window although she's never seen anyone. She doesn't like to go to the basement to get potatoes because she can't reach the light and some rotten potatoes are slimy. She's afraid to look down when she crosses bridges. She doesn't know how to swim if she should fall in.

Her favorite TV programs are horse stories, war stories, circus acts (her favorite), and *The Flintstones*. Her best friends are John and Karen, and they play house together frequently. She likes to be the mommy because she bosses and spanks the baby. She does not like to be the baby and will leave the game when she is the baby. She stated she usually dreams of horses and dreams that "Fury" will protect her. She said she always dreams about animals but no humans. She would not elaborate on this. She desires to be a "big kid" so she can get out of school and go to college. She also wants to grow older because when she is 20 she can do anything and her mother can't tell her what to do, but she says it's up to her mother whether she gets married or not. She also related when she is 16 she may go on dates—but she doesn't want to go on dates because she is afraid she'll get lost. She then related how scared she was when she once got lost in a grocery store. She looked out the window toward the end of the interview and stated that she might climb out on the roof but she was afraid she might get blown away.

Toward the end of the second hour she talked easily and without many overt signs of anxiety. However, she indicated that she wanted to terminate the session by asking several times whether she could now go out with her mother. She accepted a roll of lemon candy; she did not care to eat any there but wished to take the whole roll home. She sat quietly in the hall until her mother returned.

Case 2. Abby, age 8½ years: Abby is a dark-haired, rather pale girl of average size with slightly protruding teeth. She has a pseudomature manner, pedantically enunciating words with a rather grown-up vocabulary. She gives the appearance of the prissy "good little girl." Conversation was logical and clear but had the quality of repeating just what her mother had said. There were no reversals of pronouns. She was correctly oriented to time, place, and person. She knew she was being brought for examination because of "nervousness." She could not describe how her "nervousness" showed itself or what discomfort, if any, it caused her.

Eye contact was frequent but the relationship was distant. She moved around the room most of the time, talking rapidly in response to questions. When she would stop or sit down to talk with the examiner, there was much fidgeting of hands. High-pitched, inappropriate giggling continued throughout the hour. She was very attentive to the examiner and stayed with assigned tasks such as drawings. When asked about school,

Abby said, "School is dirty. The boys call me retarded. They put me up on a table and pulled my dress up and took pictures. Boys are dirty. The boys next door (they are 3 and 4 years old) come over just when I am napping and make noise." She has no friends. "Mother says boys are rough and boyish." There was a very lonely quality when she said, "Some girls have long hair." This statement was abruptly interjected into the conversation and seemed irrelevant to the question about friendships.

When asked about her relationship with her brother, she responded, "My brother carries me sometimes. I like to be carried all over. I'd like to be a cuddly cat; you would not be lonely and people pet you. I am the baby in the family and I'll always be the baby." Asked what she'd do when grown up, she replied, "I'll be a secretary like you (pause), oh, I'll be a doctor." There was no elaboration of this.

She denied ever getting angry except when she is "nervous." "Then I holler at the devil—dumb old idiot—then I call Mother stupid and other names. She doesn't like it" (much tense high-pitched giggling). She was evasive and vague when asked about her father, saying only that he is "nice" and they have "fun." She couldn't remember any of the activities with which they have "fun." She denied that either she or her father ever got angry and called each other names.

Abby said she spends much time daydreaming "but only of the songs Mother taught me." She talked readily and in great detail about her dreams and fantasies. Indeed, most of the spontaneous conversation consisted of telling dreams or fantasy stories. She did not clearly differentiate her stories from her dreams, making it difficult to know what she was trying to tell the examiner or to know the relevance of her conversation to the activity of the moment or her life situation. Nightmares are very real and come often and, although scary, appear to be enjoyed. "Monsters, creatures, and beings look at me, show me their teeth, and want to eat me. They chase me into the dark forest all the time very close together. They get closer and closer and it is dark as night." She then put the playroom light out with great glee. A Hansel and Gretel theme with a wicked witch was repeated often. These dreams were usually fascinating, with tall trees making everything dark. Her affect while telling these stories is best described as apprehensive yet pleasurable.

Drawings were age-appropriate but were pictures of a family and a witch's house surrounded by big trees. Wishes included (1) to be a bird "so I'd fly in the air when people chase me," (2) to have some swimming pools "so that I won't have to go to school," and (3) to go to Florida and "swim in the deep deep ocean where it will be dark." She was unable to explain the connection between having swimming pools and not going to school.

Comparison of the Mental Status of These Two Girls

Neither a nosological classification nor a diagnostic formation is possible on the basis of these mental status interviews alone. However, it should be apparent that, both quantitatively and qualitatively, Abby, the second child, demonstrates a greater degree of personality disturbance in the interview situation than Jane does.

APPEARANCE. Neither of the girls showed any outstanding abnormality or difference from each other in their general appearance.

MOOD OR AFFECT. Each of the girls was described by the examiner as appearing fearful and anxious. Both girls demonstrated excessive hand movement. Jane appeared more composed, yet more tense and inhibited. By contrast Abby seemed flighty. Abby demonstrated inappropriate affect as she discussed some of her problems and was unable to verbalize appropriate concern about her feelings. Jane made it clear that her fears were distressful to her. Although apparently too fearful (or possibly too obstinate) to move, she demonstrated both an ability and a partial desire to comply when she quickly and furtively obeyed the examiner's requests while he was out of the room.

COPING MECHANISMS. During Jane's first hour when she stood rooted to the floor, it was not possible to tell whether she was frightened or angry about the examination. Her body posture, the fact that she was willing to fulfill the examiner's requests while he was out of the room, and her subsequent telling of her many fears support the idea that she was quite frightened. She was also frightened of displeasing the teacher, of high places, of being alone, of the dark, and of growing up. At first she handled her fear by constriction and avoidance but by the second hour had overcome much of her fear of the examiner. She appeared to be trying to handle her other fears by intellectualizing in the form of reasoning logically and planning for various eventualities. None of these defense mechanisms can be considered particularly pathologic per se. However, her constriction and avoidance may well be responsible for some of her poor performance in school. She is obviously anxious, and therefore her coping mechanisms are not completely successful. Her desires to grow up and emancipate herself from her mother, while believing that her mother will handle major decisions (such as marriage), are not particularly inappropriate for an 8-year-old girl. However, if such notions persist into puberty and adolescence, we would be forced to say that her ability to comprehend adult independent functioning is impaired. Troublesome sexual and aggressive impulses are not discussed directly by Jane, but their presence is implied in her many fears and her concerns about growing up.

In contrast, Abby openly recounted fears and preoccupation with sexual and aggressive impulses. These impulses were not acted out directly during the examination. She may verbally assault her mother at times, or this could be fantasy. The fact that appropriate affect does not accompany her thoughts is considered by many clinicians to be an unconscious coping device, serving to make such thoughts psychologically tolerable. The unusual amount of fantasy in which the aggressive and sexual themes were reviewed may also be considered a coping mechanism to lessen conscious anxiety. The sexual and aggressive content of her fantasies are only thinly disguised, if at all. Unconscious phenomena cannot be observed directly but can only be inferred. One cannot be certain that the fantasy and separation of appropriate affect are attempts to cope with anything. Yet, if we accept the premise that sexual and aggressive impulses are common and highly charged human attributes, we must say that Abby is quite unusual in her expression of these feelings.

PERCEPTION AND ORIENTATION. There was no disturbance reported in orientation to time, place, or person for either of the girls. At no point was there any question abut Jane's ability to perceive reality. Although Abby does not show a profound disturbance in this area and, if pressed, might well have admitted that such things as boys' taking pictures of her genitals had not really happened, she presented these fantasies as if they were a factual answer to the examiner's question about her school adjustment. Again, when asked about her relationship with her brother, she became lost in her own desires to be petted and cuddled, leaving the listener with only the foggiest notion of her brother or what their relationship might be like. She was so absorbed in her fantasies that she showed no concern about the listener's comprehension. We were unable to get any history of molestation.

THOUGHT PROCESSES AND VERBALIZATIONS. At first Jane showed a paucity of conversation, but gradually this reached a normal level. As she improved in her ability to converse with the examiner, she demonstrated coherence, logic, and orderliness in her thinking. By contrast, Abby talked readily and in considerable volume from the very beginning. She always responded to the examiner's questions but was quickly stimulated by her own inner thoughts and would elaborate unnecessarily and irrelevantly to inquiries. The examiner did report much of her conversation to be logical and clear, but at those times she seemed to be repeating things her mother had said. Her ability to parrot adults, her appropriate drawings, and her relating of the Hansel and Gretel story indicate that Abby is capable of some conventional thinking.

FANTASY. As was indicated, Abby's fantasies are not in themselves terribly uncommon in childhood. However, they preoccupy her with such intensity that it was hard to get her to attend to other topics. The excessive number of fantasies, coupled with her preoccupation with primitive sexual and aggressive urges, are unusual in an 8-year-old girl. Even if they are not unusual, the ease with which she shares them and the apparent unawareness that such fantasy is not expected from little girls this age are pathologic. Abby did not elaborate on her three wishes, so it is difficult to understand their meaning to her. However, the unlikelihood of her wishes ever being fulfilled points again to Abby's tenuous hold on reality.

Jane did not reveal any spontaneous fantasies, and she did not play during the interview situation. However, she did tell about her play with friends in the community. Playing house is certainly a very conventional activity for an 8-year-old girl. In her particular case, the play she described seemed to be on the theme of freeing herself from adult domination by assuming the adult role, bossing and spanking the baby, and refusing to assume the role of the baby in relation to her playmates. She did not elaborate on her dreams, and this examiner does not know the significance of dreams that contain no human beings. However, the fact that Fury, a well-known horse, protects her in her dreams indicates that the dreams must have frightening content. Other wishes she gave in the course of conversation were her desire to grow up, go to college, and be free of her mother's domination. Although she fantasizes about the prospect of growing up, she also indicates that there are fears connected with growing up and being free from parents. On the basis of this interview it can be said that Jane is capable of indulging in fantasy, does not do so to excess, perhaps is somewhat constricted in this area, and did not reveal any pathologic fantasies.

SUPEREGO. In examining the child and observing her playroom behavior, it is usually much easier to discern defects in the conscience than it is to be certain she has a well-internalized concept of right and wrong. Certainly, both of these girls manifested an awareness of what society accepts as proper and improper behavior. Even Abby, who had been reported to strike out and be disruptive in school, did not indulge in any overt aggressive behavior in the playroom situation and seemed quite aware of what the adult world considers good and bad behavior. The aggressive and sexual impulses were permitted expression only in fantasy and were rationalized or presented as something beyond her control and not willfully indulged.

CONCEPT OF SELF AND OBJECT RELATIONS. Both girls appeared to appraise the role of the examiner realistically and see him as a helping individual. Jane was initially quite frightened and perhaps negativistic with the examiner, but this is not considered unusual unless it persists over many interviews. Allowance must be made for the newness of the situation. Although the examiner felt Abby was "distant" and could not always be understood, the child gave many signs of trying to establish rapport. On the basis of these observations, one would feel that neither child is completely incapable of making meaningful human relations and each has a desire for closeness with adults. Their relationships are further differentiated, however, when we look at their direct and indirect references to other people in their lives. Jane spontaneously mentioned friends with whom she apparently plays appropriately. She seems to be identified with the female role regarding growing up, completing her schooling, and getting married. She showed an ambivalent dependence upon her mother that is not very unusual. Abby has no friends that she could name. She identifies herself as being a baby and appears to have accepted this role. She was vague about her relationship with her brother and father, except as they might reinforce her baby role. She apparently sees her mother as "wicked," a stimulant of unacceptable anger and not an ego ideal. However, her quotations of her mother and her attempt at presenting herself as a prissy "good little girl" indicate some desire to fulfill her mother's expectations for her as she understands them.

Comparative Summary

Even without any consideration of the dynamics or the personal and family histories of these two children, it should be obvious that Abby is the sicker of the two youngsters. Although the interview does not show Abby to be completely out of contact with reality, conventional reality considerations influence her thinking and behavior much less than is true for Jane. Abby has a breakthrough of primitive instinctual urges. Although she showed less overt and conscious anxiety, her mechanisms of dealing with her feelings appear to be more pathologic. Her thinking tends to be tangential, as compared with Jane's, and conversation is stimulated more by her inner fantasies and impulses than by the reality situation. In the area of fantasy Abby reveals much more pathology, both qualitatively and quantitatively. In the area of object relations and identifications Abby appears to be at the level of a much younger child than Jane. There is nothing in either of these interviews to suggest that the girls have any gross impairment of intellect, and this impression was borne out by the formal intellectual assessments previously mentioned.

The mental status observations cannot establish cause or prognosis beyond question, because behavior is always multidetermined and, like headache or stomachache, may result from a variety of causes. However, these data can give clues regarding cause and outcome. Such clues can then be substantiated or refuted by the history and by other physical and psychological testing. There probably is not one specific type of behavior exhibited by either of these girls that has not been seen at one time or another in other 8-year-olds who were asymptomatic and otherwise functioning satisfactorily.

DYNAMICS OF JANE'S SYMPTOMS. Without the history of the wide discrepancy between intellectual ability and academic achievement in the case of the first child, Jane, we are at a loss to be certain whether her overall maturation process is impaired or not. She showed mild but temporary problems in the affective area. She revealed fears that are commonly a part of growing up, and she is struggling with her dependency relationship with her mother as every human being must do during her maturing years. Projective psychologic testing "revealed no sign of psychosis or even any serious neurotic disturbance." We can tentatively postulate that her fears and affective inhibitions may be unusually intense at this time and are interfering with her learning. If so, are her "normal" fears and childish obstinacy being intensified by attitudes and circumstances in the home and/or the school, or is this a temporary reaction to the growth process itself? In brief, Jane appears on examination to have all of the ego functions essential for learning, yet she is not doing so. The only other possible explanation of her school failure is some organically caused specific learning disability. Although there was no evidence of gross or "soft" neurologic signs during the mental status examination, the possibility of organically determined impairment of learning should be further explored by careful scrutiny of the developmental history and by psychologic testing. Further study failed to support any notion of an organic infirmity. However, family history revealed both parents to be shy and inhibited, with a history of problems similar to Jane's in their own school background. Father failed first grade and dropped out at grade 10. Mother completed 12 grades but with great difficulty "due to shyness." They told of sexual and other marital problems about which they do not talk. Both parents stated that the mother is overcritical and nagging toward the father, who withdraws into TV viewing. Each claimed to have found some social and vocational satisfaction "by going his own way." They continue to share the same house and the children, yet they find their marriage tolerable rather than satisfying. Both have histories of disruptive relations in their primary families, and neither parent has reached a comfortable emancipation from his own parents. The mother had been moderately punitive with Jane about poor school work and "acting so shy." At the same time she resented the teacher's labeling Jane "immature" and felt that psychiatric referral was unnecessary. The diagnostic evaluation concluded that family patterns of interacting and handling emotions are such that these individuals are not realizing their optimum potential in relation to each other and to society. However, they do not suffer any specific psychiatric disease entity. Jane's symptoms are a reaction to and a reflection of the family life. Treatment would have to be directed at improving both intellectual and affective communication among family members. Their repertoire of coping mechanisms would have to be expanded beyond their characteristic patterns of avoidance, denial, withdrawal, and obstinance. In our experience, Jane's school problem should improve with psychotherapy alone and remedial education would not be required. However, if her inhibited approach to learning continues beyond the primary grades, treatment will become more complicated.

The evaluating team could not settle on a diagnosis or come up with an explanation for Jane's poor academic performance or her many fears. It was postulated that this uncommunicating family was consciously or unconsciously withholding information, possibly out of anger at the school for making the referral or out of fear that the "delicate balance" of the family's interaction would collapse. We recommended a series of family group therapy sessions to try to help Jane with her difficulty in communicating and to further explore the reasons for Jane's poor school performance. The family agreed to this plan. After two group sessions the mother called to cancel the appointment and said that they did not care to reschedule any further appointments.

DYNAMICS OF ABBY'S SYMPTOMS. The disturbance in affect demonstrated by Abby, the second child described, is considered a sign of serious illness. Although such a finding could be a temporary reaction to severe stress, the possibility seems unlikely in this case. Abby also shows moderate to marked pathology in her perception of reality, her coping mechanisms, her use of fantasy, her thinking organization, her self-concept, and her object relationships. Empirically, we know that this number and degree of ego malfunctions are only seen in seriously ill youngsters whose maturation has been slowed for a considerable period of time or has been reversed.

The completed case study included detailed personal and family histories, physical and neurologic evaluations, and psychologic testing. The projective tests showed distortions of reality, disorganized thinking and impairment in her capacity to make empathic relationships with others. There was overwhelming evidence of a chronic pathologic interaction between mother and child since birth. Whether the pathologic process began with the mother or child cannot be settled. The pregnancy and birth were described as physically normal, but Abby was "different," more "irritable" and more "difficult," from the beginning. The mother suffered a chronic depression, which had existed in a mild to moderate degree for at least 5 years before Abby's birth. It had been hoped that the new baby might improve the mother's well-being, but her depression and many somatic complaints became worse after the delivery. Throughout infancy and preschool development, the mother-child dyad was characterized by many disappointments and frustrations, with constant battles of will and exchanges of hostility alternating with periods of remorse and intense affection and clinging by both mother and child. The father described himself as a "peace at any price" man who felt helpless to restore equanimity to his home. He was successful in his work and undertook community activities that required him to be away a great deal. He expressed affection toward and interest in Abby but was disappointed and worried. He confirmed his wife's statement that there was some "hard to define" yet definite difference in Abby from the beginning.

Abby's destructive behavior both at home and school was at times quite dangerous. On our recommendation, the parents took her to a residential treatment center for further evaluation and inpatient therapy.

EXAMINATION OF AN ADOLESCENT WHO HAD BEEN UNDER CHRONIC STRESS

By the time the child reaches adolescence, it is possible to use the more conventional adult type of interview to assess the patient's mental status. However, young people are still in the process of maturing, and the fluidity of the personality is more like a child's than an adult's. The adolescent, like the child, is also more vulnerable to environmental stress and is still under the normal pressures of the growing process itself. A "premorbid adjustment" and "specific onset of illness" seem harder to define than for adults. Hence, the degree of developmental impairment is still the *sine qua non* of the severity of illness.

Mental Status Examination

Fred, age 14 years. This patient was referred because he "has lost interest in school, going from A's and B's in fifth grade to failure in the seventh." He also has become overtly hostile to his family. Fred is a tall, slender boy who was dressed in wash pants and sport shirt, like his father. He has bangs down to his eyes, thick glasses, and dental braces. During the initial interview with his parents, Fred kept an almost constant smirk on his face, which would spread to a smile when his various misdeeds were discussed. He appeared quite hostile to both parents, referring to his mother and father as stupid, to his mother as a liar, and to his father as a coward. It was noted that he became anxious only when the interviewer asked about his father's illness. (The father suffers a chronic degenerative hereditary neurologic disorder, Huntington's Chorea). In the one-to-one interview he always referred to his parents with defiance and hostility. He avoided showing any remorse or sadness during the 4 hours he was interviewed. He was friendly and serious with the interviewer but had difficulty maintaining eye contact or showing any emotion other than hostility or self-satisfaction when misconduct was discussed.

The patient was oriented to time, place, and person. No defects in neurosensory perception were noted. Except for a slight slurring of speech, no neurologic abnormalities were observed.

His wishes were for a new bike, a go-cart, and a lawn tractor. The patient says he dreams rarely, but when he does they are pleasant dreams about playing with his friends. When asked to draw a picture of a person, he stated that he did not like to draw people and would prefer to draw something else. He did, however, draw a picture of a man who he said proceeded to make a cannon "for killing Yankees." Although Fred claimed to have many friends, he had trouble remembering their names. He could not or would not describe activities he enjoys with his friends, and he is not a member of any organized extracurricular groups. Fred fended off any suggestions that he might have problems or be depressed either by total denial or by ignoring the questions. At times he turned his attention completely to reading a newspaper he had brought to the interview. He stated that his only problems were trying to get a new bike and one particular teacher at school. He would say such things as "I don't like to think about myself" and when asked why, "because I'm too busy thinking about riding my bike and playing with my dogs."

Fred responded to every question with concrete answers but never voluntarily started the conversation. He seemed preoccupied with thoughts of weapons and violence and referred to his BB gun and large knife. In a somewhat threatening manner he told the interviewer that he was accurate in throwing his knife up to 60 feet. He also stated that he would like to have a double-barreled shotgun. His favorite play activities are swimming, riding his bike, and fighting. His vocabulary was quite adequate. He spoke matter-of-factly with no pressure but seemed to take a joy in relating events of violence, e.g., punching his sister and shooting birds.

Fred appears to have a well-developed intellectual superego in that he readily distinguishes right from wrong. However, when asked about specific misdeeds reported by his parents, he stated that these weren't his fault but were done only for "revenge."

Fred looks at himself as "a little brat." He identifies more closely with his father's illness than with his father, regards himself as "worthless," and thinks in the future he will be a burden to others. He denied much specific knowledge of his father's disease, except that it is hereditary among males. He categorically denied any concern that he has or might develop Huntington's Chorea. Fred appears to have a high-normal IQ.

Even without an item-by-item review of Fred's ego functions, it is apparent that his social and psychologic growth is impaired to a moderate degree. His maturation has slowed to the point where his progress in school and his peer relations are impaired and his relations with his family are deteriorating.

A simple explanation for his school failure might be that his knowledge of a 50–50 chance of impending neurologic disease has completely demoralized him. Even his hostility to parents, peers, and the examiner in actions as well as fantasy could be understood as an emotional response to this "impending disaster." If so, this "reaction to stress" gives us a picture of the boy's characteristic defense mechanisms.

Is this character defense specific for chorea or is it a psychologic emulation or identification with the father, who was described elsewhere in the case record as being irritable, explosive, and depressed? Depression, irritability, and impaired intellectual functioning have been considered early signs of organic deterioration that may occur several or many years before the onset of the abnormal movements in Huntington's Chorea.[3] Questions about specific etiology are thus raised by the mental status exam, but the answers depend upon further study. Neurologic examination could neither confirm or refute Huntington's Chorea, and genetic studies to settle the issue had not yet been developed.

It is sufficient for our thesis on the use of the mental status examination to say that this boy shows definite behavioral and personality abnormalities. His disturbance may be the result of either early organic brain disease or functional life-experience factors or both. Not only is he failing to progress socially and intellectually into adolescence, but his ability to cope with feelings of anger and fear seems to be regressing to the preschool level. It is impossible to remove the stress of his reality (the heredity). Therefore, psychologic therapy, if it is possible at all, must be directed at reducing fear (possibly through education about this illness); helping him suppress or redirect overt, inappropriate expressions of anger; and improving his self-image. Alienating himself from the world as he is now doing may be the only possible outcome for this child's dilemma. However, without a trial of psychotherapy I cannot accept such a prognosis. Unfortunately, Fred adamantly refused to participate in a trial of psychotherapy and his parents supported him.

SUMMARY

Mental status profiles for five different children have been presented in detail and their ego functions compared with each other. None of the children showed disturbances in every area of the personality. By qualitative and quantitative assessment of the ego functions, it is possible to estimate the depth of the illness for each child. The mental status examination gives clues regarding etiology and prognosis, but matters pertaining to cause, indicated treatment, and possible outcome must be based upon the total case study, including personal and family history, plus physical and further psychologic examinations. In the next chapters we will discuss total patient evaluations, of which the mental status examination is only one part.

REFERENCES

1. American Psychiatric Association: *Diagnostic and Statistical Manual of Mental Disorders,* 3rd Ed. Washington, D.C., 1980.
2. Kanner, L.: Early infantile autism. J. Pediat., *25*:211, 1944.
3. Rowland, L.P.: *Merritt's Textbook of Neurology,* 7th Ed. Philadelphia, Lea & Febiger, 1984.

6

EXAMINATION OF PRESCHOOL CHILDREN

It is commonly thought that preschool children are particularly difficult to examine psychiatrically because of their limited verbal ability. Our own experience has been that the vast majority of preschool patients, even as young as 2 years of age, are quite capable of verbal interchange with adults if given enough time. It is also possible to learn a great deal about a child by observing his interaction with others, his use of toys and his manipulation of his own body. Consequently, our approach with these children is essentially the same as described in Chapter 3, with appropriate modifications for the examiner's handling of the interview process.

Under ordinary circumstances, 2 or 3 hours of free play with a preschool child provides the examiner with sufficient observational data to draw a few conclusions about each subdivision of the mental status examination outline discussed in Chapter 4. One's own observations can be amplified by taking the history from the parents and by questioning the parents very specifically about motor, language and social skills achieved by the child so far. Some examiners spend little or no time directly examining preschool children and rely too heavily upon parental interpretations without questioning the data upon which the parents base their conclusions. It is important to spend time with the parents observing the child, reviewing the "baby book" plus studying old photographs and home movies. We must try to learn whether the child has had certain skills and lost them (regression) or just never achieved them at all (developmental lag).

COMMUNICATION

It is a pleasure to watch the ease with which two or three preschool children can interact and communicate. Most of us had excellent ability to communicate with 3-year-olds when we were also in our preschool years. Unfortunately, in the process of becoming an adult, social conditioning, repression, suppression and intellectualization seem to have become highly developed at the expense of our ability to enjoy social interchange with very young children. Some grown-ups do not talk with youngsters. They appear to talk *at* them or talk down to them in a patronizing way. Others, especially men, appear to be most ill at ease in relating to infants and toddlers in any except the authoritarian role. However, the ease with which a "grandfather type" communicates with preschoolers is often impressive. Perhaps he is less preoccupied with worldly matters and has more time than younger men. It is equally possible that, by the grandfather age, men are no longer afraid to display talents that society says inherently belong to females. During high school and college, many women gain experience with infants as babysitters and mothers helpers. Comparatively few men have this background.

Whatever the reasons are, it does seem that child psychiatrists in training, and many with years of experience, are very unsure of themselves when asked to examine or treat preschool children. Fortunately, this situation is changing, and an increasing number are devoting a major proportion of their professional energies to the study of preschoolers. Some training centers offer didactic instruction and supervised experience in well-baby clinics and nursery schools. In addition, the training child psychiatrist should seek every opportunity among his family and friends to care for and play with infants and toddlers. Not until one has learned to maintain his composure in the presence of runny noses, dirty pants and screaming wigglers can he be comfortable enough to observe infant behavior objectively.

COMPREHENSION PROBLEMS

The examination of preschool children poses difficulties other than communication. The ego functions that we wish to examine are still developing rapidly or have not even appeared yet. We have difficulty describing the child's behavior, let alone comprehending its meaning or significance. We know that the younger the child, the more global are his responses to both physiologic and psychologic stress. Stable behavior patterns are still developing and are extremely vulnerable to change under relatively little tension. Certain behaviors seem to reveal something about the child's biologic state or developmental level and/or reflect his current social experiences (the family). However, the child as a unique person simply cannot be described or adequately understood if separated from any knowledge of his family or his biologic development. The capacity to cope differs markedly from child to child, even at a very young age. Perhaps because clinicians are so aware of the great importance of the preschool years, we cannot help worrying about the predictive value of any of our behavioral observations.

The two crucial questions relevant to the examination of very young children suspected of delayed development are as follows: (1) Is his development at the normal level for his chronological age? (We will discuss developmental quotients later.) (2) If the child is not functioning at his age level, is the impairment temporary or not; i.e., will he catch up to his age group? The clinician must be able to tread the fine line between falsely reassuring and unnecessarily alarming the family about the child's development.

Regarding the first question on normalcy, the amount of variability within the normal range on most any developmental parameter is considerable. Many years ago Gesell[7,8] illustrated how age-specific certain classes of behavior are in normally developing children. However, in consideration of all the variables cited previously that may adversely affect the child's ability to demonstrate his true developmental level at any given time, serial observations over many months may be necessary. We need both a cross-sectional and a longitudinal view of the patient's development. Before we can say with some confidence that the child has impaired development in one or more areas and give an estimate of his chances of "catching up" with his age group, we like to have at least three examinations at 6-month intervals. If the child does not acquire age-appropriate skills in that 18 months, the parents should be advised to seek special training and special education for the child. Of course, during that 18 months, every effort should be made to correct any environmental problems that are obstructing normal development as well as to search for possible biologic causes of the developmental delay. Among the possible biologic causes, one must consider genetic factors, maternal health during pregnancy, untoward perinatal events, congenital or other illnesses, impaired perceptual functions, poor nutrition and/or almost any other health problem.

It is important to know the intactness of the auditory and visual apparatuses of all children. This is especially true for preschoolers, for the ability to see and to hear profoundly affects language development and the capacity to learn or develop many ego functions. The training clinician should take verbatim notes at every infant or toddler interview. After studying the notes of several observational sessions, it will be possible, in most instances, to provide descriptive data for each of the mental status items listed in the preceding chapter.

There are some problems, though. With the completely nonverbal child, we sometimes guess and have to say he "looks" or "seems" happy or sad. However, there is no interobserver reliability among adults observing the behavior of nonverbal children. Thought processes are often just not available or can only be implied by watching the child's play and the way he organizes it. Sometimes spontaneous play reveals at least a beginning of "awareness of problems," and sometimes it does not. Does a child's apparent concern about personal appearance reflect something about her self-concept or her relations with the parents, or both? Unless the child is profoundly disturbed, she and the diagnostician can develop many means of nonverbal communication that will enhance the examiner's ability to observe and describe the behavior, even when the child's verbal ability is very limited. Many deaf children begin spontaneously to develop some lip reading skills by the age of 2 years and are able to communicate nonverbally long before that. In fact, the child's lack of ability to attend to another person and to use facial expressions and gestures to communicate wishes along with an apparent indifference or unwillingness to try to communicate can be important findings in differentiating infantile autism (DSM-III Pervasive Developmental Disorder) from hearing impairment, mental retardation, severe negativism and withdrawal, or some form of delayed language-learning skills such as developmental aphasia. The autistic child stands out as having the most severe impairments in his ability to interact with the environment.

Some preschool children may be particularly difficult to examine if extreme fearfulness or some profound mental disturbance constricts their play or interferes with their verbal and nonverbal communication. (See the case of Bobbie M. later in the chapter.)

EARLY DEVELOPMENTAL DEVIATIONS

It is important to understand that preschool youngsters are in the midst of very rapid developmental processes that have a wide range of variability at any given age level. A 1-month lag at one examination may not be important if, at subsequent examinations, he is performing at age level. However, if skill-acquisition rate does not accelerate to bring him up to age level, we find that what was originally only a 1-month lag becomes magnified as the child grows older. Too often, the mental status, even when combined with a careful history, fails to answer the questions of parents or the examination itself raises several additional important issues. However, no longer is it necessary or desirable just to "wait and see" how he does when he enters school.

It is often, but not always, difficult to apply a diagnostic label (see Chapter 7 on nosology) to a preschool child confidently, even after extensive examinations. Most often, the issue with this age group is not to determine the presence or absence of a specific psychiatric disorder. Rather, the concerns are about developmental level compared to age expectation and the rate of development. If one is to help the very young child achieve healthy patterns of functioning, it is imperative to know the rate and direction of maturation. It is important to know in which ways a child differs from others the same age, whether these differences have the potential for adversely affecting her future and, if so, whether the differences can be expected to lessen or increase over time.

For the preceding reasons, the child psychiatrist must be taught a great deal about standardized psychologic tests for preschool children. Developmental testing skill is not easy to acquire. However, the child psychiatrist, at the very least, must know enough about preschool "norms" to make knowledgeable referrals to clinical psychologists trained in the administration of preschool tests and to use the test results intelligently in planning for the patient. In practice, most child psychiatrists probably do not administer standardized preschool tests, even if they have mastered the testing skills, because of the time-consuming nature of the tests and because their patient volume in this age group is not sufficient to keep their testing skills sharpened. The case material that follows illustrates the ways that information from standardized tests can illuminate a mental status report and formal testing can accompany the mental status data in ongoing evaluations.

It must be recognized, however, that the psychologists' examination instruments also have serious limitations. DeMyer et al.[3,4] point out that none of the "currently used standardized psychological test(s) for preschool children can come up with a reliable profile of intellectual, verbal, perceptual-motor, and motor performance over sufficiently wide mental age ranges." Some tests are useful for children less than 2½ years of age, and others can be used only at the nursery and kindergarten levels. DeMyer and her colleagues describe their developmental profile, which largely comprises items from previously standardized and well-known infant and preschool tests.

The so-called IQ tests, such as the Binet and Wechsler, were originally standardized and continue to be used with school-age children for the express purpose of predicting the child's ability to perform in the academic situation. Many mental functions necessary for school performance simply cannot be assessed at the preverbal and early verbal stages. Most investigators and clinicians believe that developmental rate and level probably are significantly related in some ways to subsequent IQ ratings. However, the exact correlations between specific developmental parameters and later academic performance factors continue to elude us.

In our society, if we erroneously label a child as "mentally retarded," we run a serious risk of sentencing the child with a self-fulfilling prophecy. However, mental retardation cannot be prevented by merely not labeling it as such. The various preschool tests can give a better estimate of the child's developmental levels than can nonstandardized clinical observations. Repeated testing at 6-month to yearly intervals can provide our only information about developmental rate. The clinician must help the parents accept that long-term study is the only method for answering their questions. After several years of trying to promote healthy development to the best of our ability in a particular child, the ultimate prognosis may become obvious.

With the present state of our knowledge, we cannot predict neurosis, delinquency, or social adaptability from a single mental status exam. However, from the family history and by continual observation, we can identify early affective, social and integrative deviations, as well as environmental phenomena known to be frequently present in the prenatal and early history of socially and psychologically maladapted individuals. When such findings are present in a preschool child, he may be considered "at risk" and treatment on both an ameliorative and preventive basis is indicated.

Mental Status Examinations of Infants and Preschoolers: Case Illustrations

THE MENTAL STATUS OF A 1-YEAR-OLD

Name: K.C.

K.C. is a 13½-month-old male who was burned when he knocked over an ironing board, causing the iron to fall on the dorsum of his left hand, leaving second- and third-degree burns to the third, fourth and fifth digits. He was transferred from another hospital for excision of the burned area and preparation for grafting. The child was seen for psychiatric consultation as part of an ongoing study[13] of the psychiatric sequelae of severe burns. Because of isolation and sterile techniques, all burned children are examined in their own room on the Burn Unit and the examiners are required to wear gowns, masks and sterile gloves.

K.C. was always noted to be active on the unit. He was pleasant, affectionate and gregarious. He continuously explored any area permitted but, when told he could not go beyond a certain point, he would stop traveling and return on command. He had good eye contact and spontaneously used some intelligible single words. He would not repeat words after the examiner but said *ball* when he was shown one and the examiner said it at the same time. He hugged a stuffed toy and rolled a truck on the floor when these were presented. He was shown a small car and then the car was quickly placed under the sheet. He searched for it. He continuously reached for objects that were beyond his arm's length, and, when offered a stick, he would retrieve the toy. He walked without assistance, using his arms in the balance role. He was noted to be affectionate with peers as well as adults. At no time did there appear to be any evidence of depression or withdrawal. Appetite was good and there was no disturbance in sleep pattern. The nurses liked the child and had no complaints about him.

When E. asked K.C. to show his slippers, he lifted one foot. When offered a mirror, he smiled and patted it but did not identify himself in the mirror as an older child would do. He pointed to his hair and eyes when asked, but did not identify any other parts of the body. K.C. played patty cake, but did not hold up a hand or index finger in imitation of the examiner when asked to. He was able to pick up and release the soft sponge ball and, when requested, released it toward the examiner from his seated position. While standing up upon request, he would crudely thrust the ball forward, toddling both before and after the throw. He could not catch the ball as an older child would. He picked up with his thumb and index finger a "fruit loop" (cereal) that was offered to him, but he could not unwrap a small piece of candy. He intently watched the examiner scribble with a crayon on a piece of paper but was unable to hold adaptively or use the crayon himself. When presented with a colored ring stack, he removed one ring and then removed all of the rings on request but was unable to place them back on the stick. He was offered some small blocks and, upon request, placed one block in a cup and then placed all of them in the cup. He could imitate a two-block tower but could not stack any more blocks when requested to do so.

A complete personal developmental and family history was obtained from the parents. All indications are that there were no problems regarding K.C. during pregnancy, delivery or the first year of life, and he seems to be a happy, well-functioning member of a well-integrated family. The burn incident appeared to be a true accident, which happened during a visit to the grandmother's house. She had left the ironing board, forgetting to turn off the iron.

Discussion

K.C. certainly appeared to be socially at his age level in his interactions with other people and his investigative response to a new environment. He had a memory appropriate to his age, demonstrated by his searching for the hidden toy and his spontaneous imitation of sounds. (We would not expect him to be able to repeat words after the examiner for another 8 or 10 months.) His use of the mirror was satisfactory for a 1-year-old, as was his ability to identify at least two parts of his own body. His reaching out for toys and his use of the stick to obtain those beyond his arm's length are behaviors commonly seen at around 15 or 17 months. His ability to inhibit an activity on command and showing his slippers when asked indicate 10- to 15-month-old behavior. His method of walking was appropriate for 1 year of age, as was his use of the soft ball. His inability to catch the ball was not significant, since we would not expect that for another year and a half or so. His use of his thumb and finger (pincer-grasp) and his patty cake are skills that should be achieved somewhat before 1 year of age. For his age, he should have been able to use a crayon better than he did. Whether this was negativism or the fact that one hand was bandaged is unknown. We were unable to tell whether K.C. was right- or left-handed. His use of the ring stack and his use of the small blocks indicate a 14- and 15-month-old developmental level. K.C. will be followed for a year or more by the Plastic Surgery Department and as part of the psychiatric study of burned children. However, from this mental status examination, there was no reason to suspect any personality or developmental problems so far, and this evaluation was reinforced by the Social Service family assessment.

MENTAL STATUS EVALUATION OF A 32-MONTH-OLD GIRL WITH SEVERE GLOBAL DEVELOPMENTAL DELAY

Name: Debbie D.

The child was referred by the local Welfare Department and their primary care physician "to have tests made to see why she is not talking or walking." (Welfare hopes to prepare this child for preschool in the next 4 to 5 months.)

Pregnancy and delivery normal

3 to 4 months: Rolled over

6 months: Was talking and had about 12 words by 18 months. At 1 year, the physician checking-up questioned whether the child had a hearing problem. An ear-nose-throat consultation appointment was not kept by the mother. (The mother's report of a 12- to 18-word vocabulary may be inaccurate. However, some developmentally retarded children do acquire early a small vocabulary that is largely echolalic. They may not learn to use the words meaningfully and the vocabulary subsequently drops out. One can check this out by having the parents write down every word they ever heard the child say and then obtaining a description of the way the child used the words, i.e., whether she used them in association with appropriate persons, objects or actions.)

14 to 18 months: Began trying to crawl with difficulty.

20 months: Parents divorced. Debbie very close to father. Since divorce, says only "dada" when father is present.

23 months: Half-brother born. Debbie "insisted" on having her bottle back. In spite of good appetite, mother still gives her the bottle whenever she is fussy (age 32 months).

24 months: Primary care physician recommended admission to the hospital for complete developmental assessment. Mother did not follow recommendations because she was "afraid of the results" (reasons unclear from the chart).

Mother's Attitude

In spite of her fearfulness, the mother seemed concerned and cooperative. She seemed open to the idea that either physical or psychologic causes may underlie the developmental delay. She was not depressed. She welcomed paternal visitations. She was pleased about the Welfare Department's referral to the local developmental program. Mother had had "horrifying fantasies" regarding possible diagnoses, such as "brain dying," "holes in the brain," "defects in the backbone," "mental deficiency" or "the child turning into a vegetable."

Mental Status Examination

Debbie was interviewed in her hospital room along with her mother. In the beginning, she sat on her mother's lap, sucking milk out of a bottle. She angrily hit and pulled at the nipple several times. It appeared that she had been crying earlier, and tears were still rolling down her cheeks. She looked at the examiner but did not smile. The mother put her down and the child attempted to walk a few steps at mother's repeated request and reassurance that she could do so. Her gait was broad-based and she held her arms out in the balance position. (Holding the arms in this position is typical for the child just learning to walk at 10 to 14 months).

Some developmental tests were attempted. On the Denver Developmental Test, she performed at the 11- to 16-month age level, more than 16 months below her actual age of 32 months.

The Alpern-Boll Profile revealed the following: physical age, 10 months; self-help age, 14 months; social age, 20 months; academic age, 14 months: communication age, 12 months.

Other developmental tasks: She could not or would not imitate words, a task usually possible at about 13 months of age. When shown a small spoon, she did not search for it after it had been hidden under the edge of the table. She has some receptive language, in that she turned her head in response to her name, as a child well below 6 months of age can do. However, she could not, or would not, show any piece of her clothing when requested. She did respond to minor requests, such as attempting to walk at the mother's appeals. With the doll, she played appropriately for a child less than 1 year but could not follow directions to do things with the doll as an 18-month-old might.

Regarding her speech, she laughed and squealed like a child less than 6 months, but there was no repetition of two-syllable sounds (*mama, dada*) although the mother reported that she says "dada" when her father is present, a task that most children have accomplished at about 1 year of age or before.

Regarding her motor abilities, her walking was at about the 12-months-of-age level, and she could walk very little without falling (a task usually accomplished by 18 months). The child crawled on the floor but would not attempt to creep up some small steps. In ball play, she could pick it up and release it like a child before the age of 9 months, and she did purposefully release the ball to the examiner whe requested (13-month age level). She could not cast the ball from a standing position, even leaning against her mother, and she made no attempt to catch it. On hand and finger imitation, she could patty cake (9 months) and hold up her hand upon request (15 months) but could not imitate the examiner's holding up one or two fingers, as most 2- or 2½-year-olds can. Debbie could transfer an object from one hand to the other, a task that many 6-month-olds spontaneously do, but seemed to have difficulty and required much concentration. She did demonstrate the pincer grasp of the 11-month-old but could not unwrap a piece of candy or unscrew a jar lid as a 1½- or 2-year-old child can.

The child's baby pictures were reviewed. It did appear that she was sitting alone by about 8 months. In the pictures she seemed visually engaged with objects and people. There was not a single picture in which the child was seen standing on her own without support.

Discussion

The child appeared developmentally delayed in her ability to perceive and remember objects, in her receptive and expressive language and in gross and fine motor tasks. Not only were there severe impairments in language and motor abilities, but her performance on perceptual-motor tasks was extremely low compared with her chronologic age.

The mother's concern about the child's walking was certainly very realistic. In normal development, she should have been able to walk on a broad-base gait without holding her arms out like a beginner and without falling by age 18 months. Most children have developed heel-to-toe gait and some ability to run without falling by 2 years of age.

The normal developing child can say "dada" and "mama" in reference to the appropriate parent by 1 year. By the age of 18 months, most children can repeat perhaps six words, such as *ball, kitty, eat.* Repetition of two words together and the ability to say one's first name or nickname should appear shortly before the second birthday, and the repetition of two- to three-word phrases spontaneously usually appears between 2 and 3 years of age. Until the third birthday, there is wide variability in speech development, and one may not be very concerned about the delayed development if there is evidence of comprehension and normal development in other areas. At 32 months, Debbie's apparent limited comprehension and her delayed development in both visual and verbal memory, the limited receptive speech and lack of expressive speech, along with her very low levels in gross motor and fine motor performance, gave cause for genuine concern. She was also performing at a low level on the few perceptual-motor tasks that were assessed. On the basis of the preceding information, one would have to consider the following differential possibilities: hearing impairment, mental retardation, childhood onset pervasive developmental disorder and developmental aphasia.

The Audiology Department reported with "reasonable certainty" that there was no hearing impairment evidenced on the infant hearing test. For the differential of mental retardation and the pervasive developmental disorders the reader should consult the *1980 Diagnostic and Statistical Manual III.*[1]

Fear of error and the "self-fulfilling prophecy" danger makes many clinicians reluctant to offer an exact intelligence quotient for preschool children. Even so, in a child as severely impaired as Debbie, it would be unkind to withhold the diagnosis or to offer false hope to her family. A developmental quotient, ([mental age/chronological age] × 100) can be estimated and this information shared with the parents. For Debbie remedial measures have, unfortunately, already been considerably delayed. On the Alpern-Boll Developmental Profile and several of the DeMyer items, Debbie's developmental quotients (DQ) ranged from a low of 30 to a high (social age) of 60. She was performing in the retarded range in all areas. (Average DQ is 90 to 110.)

Remedial measures were indicated without further waiting or additional testing. The prognosis for near normal functioning seems very doubtful. However, it should be emphasized that we cannot say whether or not she will stay at such a low level. Additional annual testing will provide subsequent DQs by which we can assess her response to remedial procedures and, eventually, provide a long-range prognosis. The DQ is not synonymous with the IQ, but it does give a fair estimate of the degree of retardation and can be used to measure progress (developmental rate).

Debbie will be enrolled in a developmental training program near her home and followed with her family, to try to learn the causes and get some more exact concept of the prognosis before she enters nursery school or kindergarten. From the history, one must consider the possibility that the divorce and the ensuing disruption of the living situation may be contributing to the clinical picture seen at age 32 months. However, it seems that significant developmental delays were present almost from the beginning. Whatever the true facts are, it will be important for this mother to have help in establishing a stable home life for this child's continued development to whatever level her native abilities might be.

MENTAL STATUS OF A HIGHLY DISTURBED 3½-YEAR-OLD BOY

Name: Bobbie M. and twin sister, Barbie M.

The children live with their 23-year-old mother and 14-month-old half-brother. Parents separated and divorced 2½ years before Bobbie was referred. Bobbie was hospitalized 3 months prior to the referral "to give the mother a rest and to evaluate for possible seizure disorder."

Mother's Description of the Problem

"Bobbie has spells where he is completely uncontrollable. He runs in circles, throws himself into the wall head first, has bloody noses and vomits. He complains of headaches and stomachaches. I try to physically hold him and can't. He takes a lot out on the other twin and on the baby, hitting, kicking and biting. He screams the whole time. He also has a lot of trouble sleeping."

Psychiatric Examination

Bobbie was seen for three 1-hour sessions in the clinic. On the first visit, after a brief get-acquainted session with his mother and the social worker, the examiner decided to take Bobbie to the playroom. He was very reluctant to leave his mother, clinging to her and beginning to cry big tears. The examiner picked up the child and carried him to the playroom. He continued to protest verbally "No, no, no" but clung to the examiner as closely as he had to his mother, in a strong physical embrace. The examiner had some difficulty disengaging him and placing him in a chair. Once in the chair, he sat relatively immobile and continued to cry without tears for approximately 10 minutes. He finally quieted and seemed to show interest in his surroundings. An attempt was made to engage him in some of the games and tasks used in developmental testing. However, he became quite active throughout the remainder of the session, often moving about in the chair, on the floor and going from object to object in the room. He would not pay attention to explanations and requests, and it was difficult to get his attention unless the examiner repeated instructions several times. There were times when he appeared to concentrate for a short time and perform relatively well, then he would suddenly lose interest and refuse to return to the items presented. An example was the color matching rings, which at first interested him and later he rejected. He refused to try to do things such as skip or toss a ball. When left on his own, he went from item to item in the room. He did not avoid the examiner, but it was difficult to engage him in activity of any kind. It was possible to engage him briefly in the game of assigning arms and legs to a person's figure, but he had much difficulty concentrating, became easily frustrated and then refused to perform at all. By the end of the hour, his general activity was considerably less than at the beginning, and he returned calmly to his mother in the waiting room but did not greet her verbally or by touch.

At the second visit, Bobbie's twin sister, Barbie, was brought at the examiner's request, and an attempt was made to test the developmental skills of these two individuals at the same time. There was marked difference between them. Barbie listened to instructions, sat quietly in her chair and did not move unless given permission, throughout the entire session. She could be seen "processing her tasks"; i.e., she paid very close attention and seemed to study the situation before performing. In contrast, Bobbie paid little attention to any of the materials presented and performed frequently in an indifferent, if not entirely negativistic, manner. Bobbie moved about the room and in his chair and was constantly dropping items on the floor that he, himself, would jump off the chair to retrieve. Barbie seemed aware of Bobbie's difficulty and almost always would attempt to help him perform the task properly. Several times it was necessary to request that she let Bobbie make his own decisions and do the task the way he wanted. Bobbie did pay attention to Barbie's performance and needed to touch all of the items that were presented to her. Barbie had a relatively long attention span and would work until she was presented with something she could not do. Bobbie, on the other hand, very quickly became frustrated and would give up easily at a point that often seemed much below the limits of his ability. Both during the presentation of developmental tasks and in free play, Barbie seemed rather protective of Bobbie and he seemed to enjoy her attention.

On the third visit, Bobbie was seen in the playroom with his mother. He came to the room actively hitting his mother. She allowed this behavior to continue but then held his hands, at which point he began to twist and manipulate her fingers. The examiner removed Bobbie from his mother and placed him in a chair, instructing him he could leave the chair if he did not hit his mother. At that point, he began to cry loudly but did not leave his chair. His crying was ignored, but it continued unabated for 8 minutes and then tapered off completely. After he stopped crying, he began to spit, accumulating saliva on his chin and directing it indiscriminately about the room. Several times his mother admonished him not to spit, but he did it anyway. An attempt was made by the mother and the examiner to ignore his behavior as he wandered about the room, but he continued to be aggressively intrusive, both verbally and physically, especially toward his mother. The overactivity and the attention-getting devices directed at the mother never ceased completely but had lessened considerably and were not particularly bothersome during the last 15 minutes of the hour.

Comparison of the Developmental Levels of Bobbie and Barbie

(The test items used were the "Profile for Pre-School Children" compiled by Marian K. DeMyer, M.D., from 14 different standardized developmental and intellectual tests.)

Item	Bobbie	Barbie
Test Behavior Chronological age 42 months	Took two sessions for completion of items; fidgety, overactive, short attention, uncooperative	Completed items in one session; attentive, poised, sat quietly, cooperatively
Intellectual Tasks Visual Memory (picture memory)	42 months	43 months
Verbal Memory (repetition of words, digits and sentences)	Ignored instructions; silly, giggling; would not repeat any word requested	48 months
Self-awareness (identification of body parts)	42 months	48 months
Problem solving with objects	54 months	54 months
Problem solving with numbers	42 months	36 months
Language Receptive (Peabody Picture Vocabulary)	35 months	40 months
Expressive	Would not attempt to answer any questions; purposefully fell off chair and wiggled on floor	32 months
Motor Skills Gross movements, lower extremities	Would not perform any task requested but on observation of free play spontaneously showed skill at or above 46 months	54 months
Integration (ball play)	Refused directions. Skills could not be scored	48 months

Item	Bobbie	Barbie
Fine motor skills, upper extremities	Refused directions Spontaneous activities showed skills at least at the 36-month level	43 months
Perceptual Motor Skills Geometric figures	Used crayon adaptively and imitated lines and strokes up to 24 months' level and then refused to cooperate	36 to 45 months
Fit and assemble objects	36 months	48 months
Perceptual ability Color	43 months	54 months
Form	37 months	36 months

Discussion:

The main purpose of these examinations was to learn Bobbie's developmental level or mental age and, if possible, ascertain ways to treat this very unhappy and disturbed little boy. On the various test items, Bobbie's mental age varied from "unscorable" to 54 months. In the areas where a mental age could be scored, his developmental quotient (DQ = $\frac{MA}{CA} \times 100$) ranged from 83 on receptive language to 129 on problem solving with objects. Barbie's mental age ranged from 32 months on expressive language to 54 months in gross motor skills, problem solving with objects and color perception. An average DQ would not be particularly useful at this age. We noted that her lowest DQ (expressive language) was 76 and her highest (on three items) was 129. The use of a DQ score is important because, at subsequent testing, we not only wish to know the amount of increase in mental age but whether or not the improvement has brought the child any nearer to the average for his/her chronological age. An average DQ is 90 to 110.

It is obvious that Barbie was functioning at or above her age level of 42 months in most areas. Her low scores in expressive language and ability to perceive form should be double-checked in 6 months to 1 year. If the low scores are still present, she should have more definitive testing of language and intelligence some time before she enters first grade. At first glance, Bobbie seems to be functioning at a significantly lower level than his sister. However, when the examiner was able to score him in certain areas by watching his spontaneous play, he often received a score equal to Barbie's. One can speculate that his negativism and uncooperativeness lowered his developmental test scores. However, it is also possible that his inability to perform certain tasks produced considerable frustration and negativism. Many very young children become acutely upset, withdrawn or negativistic when pressured to do tasks they cannot perform well. One cannot safely use Bobbie's highest scores to estimate his overall intelligence since high variability can be the hallmark of brain dysfunction as well as emotional disturbance. Attention is part of intelligence. In this instance, it would be pseudoscientific double talk to say that his MA scores were depressed because of poor attention, especially at the point where the cause(s) of his distractibility were uncertain. Retesting a few months later, when and if the behavior and ability to relate improve, will be necessary to decide his actual mental age with more certainty.

Diagnostically, Bobbie presents the picture of both "Attention Deficit Disorder with Hyperactivity" and "Conduct Disorder, Socialized, Aggressive" (DSM-III 314.01 and 312.23). A complete family evaluation (see Chapter 9 for description of the elements of a full case study) and further observations supported both diagnoses. A trial of treatment, including a major tranquilizer and behavior modification with intensive instruction of the mother in operant principles and behavior control techniques, was instituted. Ritalin had been prescribed by another therapist in the past "without effect." In 7 or 8 weeks, dramatic improvement occurred in the form of lengthened attention span, reduced overactivity, improved sleeping patterns and an increase in compliance behavior. Verbal and physical outbursts ceased, although limit testing and some noncompliance continued. As Bobbie improved the treatment emphasis shifted, with less time being spent on techniques for controlling Bobbie's behavior and more time focused on the mother's personal problems in self-concept, as well as her mild, chronic depression. Meanwhile, Bobbie was seen in individual therapy in an attempt to uncover the thoughts and feelings underlying his negativistic and destructive behavior. Improvement was fairly steady and he did well in a "Headstart" nursery school.

The mother had given his prescribed Mellaril rather sporadically, so it had been discontinued some time before termination of regular treatment sessions. It was impossible to show whether Ritalin had had any effect on his behavior or not. At the time of termination of therapy some 2 years after the original evaluation, the therapist rated the improvement as only moderate. She (therapist) described the mother as extremely dependent, with considerable pent-up anger. Mother still had problems with limit setting and discipline. "A future crisis could upset the balance." Mother was still blaming people and situations outside the home for Bobbie's behavior.

Fourteen months later the mother returned, requesting neuropsychologic testing for possible "dyslexia" in Bobbie. There was no indication for this and she and Bobbie were invited to resume therapy. She adamantly refused.

One year later (patient now 6 years old) mother returned, bringing Bobbie; his twin, Barbie; a brother 2 years younger; and a new stepfather, whom she had married 1 year before. Bobbie had been placed in special classes for the emotionally disturbed. The new stepfather had been diagnosed as having a progressive incurable neurologic disorder and was becoming paralyzed. (We suspected but could not confirm that he suffered from Huntington's Chorea.) The family was chaotic, and all of the children were aggressive and undisciplined.

Retesting of Bobbie was extremely difficult because of severe negativism and violent outbursts. The testing showed him to have average intelligence and he was achieving academically at the appropriate grade level for his age. There was no learning disability. Projective testing did not show overt signs of psychosis. However, reality testing was quite poor and the examiner felt he was at high risk for decompensation under stress. The diagnoses of "Attention Deficit and Conduct Disorder, Socialized, Aggressive" were reconfirmed.

Over the following 2 years Bobbie received individual and group therapy plus some therapeutic camping along with major tranquilizing medication. This medication was later changed to imipramine, to which he seemed to respond better. Mother has again entered individual psychotherapy. The stepfather deteriorated mentally, became abusive and had to be removed from the home. Bobbie was gradually "mainstreamed" to the regular second grade classes and continues to learn. However, his adjustment remains tenuous in school and, at times, he is extremely infantile and dependent upon his mother. Placement for inpatient residential treatment has been considered several times and still remains a possibility. His siblings show a much better adjustment than he does.

CONGENITAL DEFORMITIES AND DEVELOPMENTAL DEVIATION

Children who suffer both serious physical and psychologic deviations or stresses early in life are most challenging from the diagnostic and prognostic viewpoint. An example of such a case is reviewed next.

Name: R.T.
Birth Date: 9/21/69   *Age:* 27 months

PRESENTING PROBLEM

"Head banging, rejecting, slow development"

HISTORY

R. was made a ward of Z. County shortly after birth. History of the natural parents is unavailable. He usually resides in a temporary foster home in his local county 200 miles from the Medical Center. He has a congenital cleft lip and palate. Following each of three surgical corrections he has convalesced in the home of Mrs. N. in this city.

Mrs. N. and the plastic surgeon requested psychiatric consultation because of R's slow development in communication, rejecting attitudes toward others, and head banging. Mrs. N. reports that the child's personality changed markedly during his last stay in his hometown. He now shows negativism toward her and refuses to eat solid foods. In spite of R.'s obvious good nutrition, Mrs. N. expressed great concern that the welfare department may take R. and other foster children from her if they do not eat properly. She naively revealed her practice of mixing vitamins and nutrients in milk and giving R. a bottle with a large-hole nipple prior to bringing him to the table for his solid foods. She seemed alarmed at the suggestion the bottles be discontinued. (Mrs. N. has been previously evaluated in this clinic upon referral of another of her foster children. Child Guidance Case #R-9156.)

MENTAL STATUS OF CHILD

R. is a fair-skinned boy with multiple bruises. He initially relates very poorly, backing away from the interviewer, and going into rocking behavior, back and forth and side to side on his feet. By the end of an hour he will interact, sit on the interviewer's lap, show a social smile, sometimes laugh when others in the room do, as well as play ball and use toys with the interviewer. He shows some spontaneous interest in toys. Behavioral observations include the following:

Plays ball for a few throws, rolling ball on floor to interviewer
Kisses rag doll
Clumsily turns toy telephone dial to produce ringing
Does not come when called or when arms offered
Sits pliantly on lap or allows self to be held

Sometimes responds to name
Vocal sounds below 8- or 9-month level, no speech or pseudospeech
Interest in toys and objects usually short
Much releasing and throwing behavior
Maintains rocking behavior for long periods
Able to stoop and pick up large ball
Infantile grasp
Laughs at some play with interviewer (ball)

R. is very pliable and compliant to physical manipulation. Spontaneous action is much lower than normal. He showed much resistance to Mrs. N.'s overtures to him during the interview. Interviewer was related to somewhat more positively. Foster mother says child relates poorly and screams when being touched by the rest of her family, except 18-month-old grandchild, who also is the only person who can get the child to laugh.

PSYCHOLOGICAL STUDY, 27 MONTHS

R. is a 2-year-old boy who was seen to determine his level of intellectual and social functioning.

He is a rather unattractive-looking child, his face disfigured by a recent operation; his arms were in splints to prevent his handling the scar. He made no protest at being taken to the interview room, and, in fact, his only visible acknowledgement of my presence was to allow me to take his hand. This lack of social contact with his environment was very characteristic of his behavior during this meeting. He never smiled or responded interpersonally with me. When I told him to look me in the eyes, he did not seem to hear. He was willing to sit up in my lap but showed no affect in this position. When left to himself, R. rocked back and forth on his feet in a repetitive self-stimulating manner.

The following are brief descriptions of R.'s behavior during this meeting: was not able to hold crayon to draw; did not immediately attend to bell that was rung by his left ear; showed no signs of imitation; did not respond to verbal commands; was able to pick up block and find rattle that had been hidden under a box; produced no recognizable language, although did make gurgling noises; motor movements generally slow and jerky; enjoyed picking up an object, throwing it, and then retrieving it. These observations of R.'s behavior could be summarized by saying that he is quite retarded in areas of language and motor and social development. However, a Vineland Social Maturity Scale was obtained from R.'s foster mother of 6 months. Although there is reason to suspect the accuracy of some of this woman's responses, her information indicated that R. has a social maturity age level between 11 months and 1 year. He is thus functioning 1 year below his age level or has a DQ near 50.

SUMMARY OF R.'S EVALUATION AT
2 YEARS, 3 MONTHS (27 mos.)

This child is approximately 1 year below his chronological age in intellectual and social development. In addition, he shows signs of emotional tension such as social withdrawal, rocking behavior, excessive crying, negativism, passivity, head banging and refusal to eat solid foods.

It is not possible to state at this age how much his delayed development is due to low native intellectual ability and how much is secondary to his emotional state.

His foster mother is extremely well-meaning and interested. However, she is a very tense, anxious person for a variety of reasons and gives the rather typical picture of the overprotective mother. Although it would be unfair, and not substantiated by objective data, to say that Mrs. N. is in any way the cause of the delayed development, it is our impression that her tenderheartedness, personal anxiety and overprotectiveness make it seem doubtful that she can give the child the calm environment and the gently persuasive training he needs to help him become more sociable and learn to do things for himself. The Occupational Therapy Department at this hospital evaluated this child last May, and Mrs. N. has not had any success with the techniques they recommended for improving R.'s behavior.

RECOMMENDATIONS

1. Transfer to a calmer home, preferably as a permanent placement. This may not be *the* answer for R., but it is certainly worth trying at this point.
2. This child, in our judgment, should be adopted only if the prospective parents are fully aware of his uncertain developmental potential. His chances of reaching an average developmental level are very questionable. They should also be aware of the genetic risk of cleft palate offspring of this child.
3. His placement in a foster or adoptive home should be with parents who are very patient, do not have high expectations or drive toward training the child, yet can exert gentle, continuous pressure for R. to learn to eat solid foods and perform other self-help and social tasks.
4. Reevaluate his mental state in 6 months.

DIAGNOSIS

Undetermined—definite slow development

PSYCHOLOGICAL STUDY, REEVALUATION, AGE 31½ MONTHS
(4½ mos. after last evaluation)

R. has been in a new foster home for the last 2 months. He is much less anxious and withdrawn than he was during the previous evaluation, although he still is not producing any intelligible language. He is currently able to respond interpersonally in that he will make eye contact and will roll a ball back and forth to another person. It was felt that R. is still probably functioning in the retarded range, but formal testing was not deemed feasible at this time.

It is recommended that R. be reevaluated in 6 months, at which time it may be possible to assess more accurately the degree of retardation present in this boy. In addition, speech therapy is recommended in the hopes of stimulating language behavior.

REEVALUATION, AGE 37½ MONTHS
(1 year after initial evaluation)

R., now age 3 years, 1½ months, was brought by his foster parents for reevaluation of his developmental level, as requested by our department, and for a follow-up appointment in Plastic Surgery. R. has been in this foster home for 8 months, and it is considered a permanent placement.

OBSERVATIONS OF THE CHILD

Comparing R. with previous examinations last May and 12 months ago, he has made a number of gains, particularly in the area of sociability. He was noted still to rock from one side to the other while standing on his feet, but this was minimal as compared to 1 year ago. He separated from his foster mother without a reaction. However, she soon came after him, saying she thought he should be taken to the bathroom first, and, on the second separation, he cried and was obviously angry at being separated from her.

In the playroom, he at first rejected all toys. He made a whining "ma" or "mama" sound as he went to and looked searchingly at the playroom door. However, he soon settled down and I was able to get a good bit of eye contact and nonverbal communication from him. I was unable to get any intelligible speech other than the "mama," but he would take my hand or make gestures for the things he wanted. For example, he could not figure how to get the doors open on a big truck after I had shown him three times. He would close the doors and then come and get my hand for me to open them again for him. When I insisted he could open the doors himself, he did so and seemed extremely pleased. He then played for a while, repeating the opening and closing of the doors to the truck. He would be easily frustrated if they did not open immediately and cried briefly. Episodically, he would stop his play and go to the door, apparently searching for his mother. He understood simple directions and obeyed me.

After briefly rolling some trucks around the floor, he climbed into the sand box and played there as a 1- to 1½-year-old child would do. He would pat and hit the sand, run it through his fingers and would pick it up with the sand on the back of his hands. He briefly paid attention to the toys in the sand box, but most of the time was spent running his hands through the sand. He then began to throw sand but stopped when I asked him to. He then engaged in some teasing behavior in which he would pick up some sand and gesture as if to throw it, look at me and then giggle when I told him not to. He still mouths toys and he tried to eat the sand. In general, he was much more friendly and sociable with me. He rejected my attempts to get him to use crayon or pencil.

Unfortunately, at the time R. was seen, the clinic was not formally recording developmental quotients. Had this been done, we might have been able to say with more certainty whether his improved skills indicated that he was catching up with his age norms or not. The overall impression was, however, that R. remained seriously retarded.

INTERVIEW WITH THE PARENTS

The parents were seen together with their social worker. These parents have a great deal of positive involvement with R. and are extremely pleased with his development. They would like to believe that the improvement of the last 6 or 8 months means that he is intellectually normal. The mother reported that he is now feeding himself; able to drink from a glass; engages in emotional interaction with the family as well as with other children; can say "Mama," "Dad" and "Hi"; and is toilet trained. He is attending a nursery school 2½ hours per day, 5 days per week and also receiving speech therapy at this school (a school report has been requested). The foster parents intend to adopt this child when he has completed his surgery for his cleft lip.

SUMMARY AND RECOMMENDATIONS AT AGE 37½ MONTHS

R. has made considerable progress, particularly in the social and human interaction area, but has not made much progress in his speech development. His play behavior and play interests still appear to be those of a child between 18 months and 2 years of age. He is toilet trained and is able to understand and usually to follow directions. He appears to this examiner to be a much more relaxed and comfortable child than he was a year ago. However, his development remains in the severely retarded range.

The foster parents were told that we strongly suspect this child is mentally retarded. At this point, he performs at the severely retarded level, but we cannot predict the upper limits of his developmental potential. R. will be hospitalized for surgery in 2 months. We have requested that he be admitted to the hospital 3 days early for a prolonged period of observation and another attempt to do standardized developmental tests on him.

PSYCHOLOGICAL STUDY, AGE 40 MONTHS

Attempted Cattell Infant Intelligence Scale and Alpern-Boll Developmental Profile.

REFERRAL

R. was seen for reassessment of his social and intellectual development. Initial evaluation at age 27 months indicated that R. was approximately 1 year below his chronological age in intellectual and social development. Additionally, signs of emotional tensions were noted in this child as he engaged in excessive crying, rocking behavior, passivity, withdrawal and head banging. Later evaluations reported a steady decrease in emotional behaviors along with an increase in the level of social responsivity. The present study was initiated as an attempt to further clarify this child's intellectual development.

BEHAVIOR NOTES

R. separated from his parents to go to the examining room with no protest. He did indicate, by his initial coolness toward the examiner and by short glances back toward his parents, that he would have preferred to stay on the ward with them. At times during the examining hour he actually would go to the door, sometimes pulling the examiner with him, and say "Mama." These behaviors are of note because of the extreme passivity this youngster exhibited in the past.

R. spent most of the hour moving about the room, going in and out of the door or walking up and down the hall. It was impossible to engage his interest in a task, a toy, or other activity for more than just a few seconds. He would respond to verbal directions but there was no sustained effort in his responses. No rocking or similar activity was noted during the hour. R. indicated his awareness of the examiner throughout the period. For instance, he would never wander very far away and would return quickly if the examiner were out of his sight.

TEST RESULTS, AGE 40 MONTHS

Items of the Cattell Scale were administered. The results were so variable, however, that no scoring was attempted. On many of the items that he did not pass, it was impossible to tell whether he was unable to do the task or simply would not put out sufficient effort to complete it. Some of the activities that he did engage in were as follows:

1. Responded to and carried out some simple commands
2. Picked up cubes and placed them in a cup
3. Built a tower out of three or more blocks
4. Scribbled spontaneously with a pencil

Generally, R. did not succeed on any of the items above the 2-year level but *seemed* capable of completing many tasks below that level. The Developmental Profile Assessment, based on maternal report, places R.'s general developmental level at about 14 months below his chronological age. The social level was his relatively highest area, but, it should be noted, this does not reflect the "emotional" quality that is a part of his social behavior (short attention, etc.). R.'s communicative (most particularly verbal) skills were not only much below age level but also significantly below R.'s own general level of development.

CONCLUSIONS

R. T.'s mental status appears to be showing continued improvement since he was initially evaluated. Social responsive behaviors are apparently on the increase while many emotional behaviors (i.e., rocking, head banging, etc.) are decreasing. Additionally, he has achieved many self-help skills such as self-feeding and undressing and can indicate his desire to use the toilet and does so with few accidents. He does make some response to simple verbal directions.

The present data indicate that R. is still approximately 1 year behind in general and intellectual development. Any predictions about his later intellectual abilities must yet be considered as tentative. The best *guess* of this examiner, at this time, is that R. will be able to go to school, but he will have to be in classes for the "trainable" rather than the "educable" retarded children. The lack of language portends a bad prognosis. Again, annual assessments are indicated to monitor his development and to advise the guardians in planning his future.

RECOMMENDATIONS

1. It seems apparent that R.'s foster parents are providing very much the kind of day-to-day home environment that R. needs. That is, they seem to combine the warmth and personal respect R. deserves with the gentle firmness that he needs. Without this firmness, R. is likely not to engage in many of the activities that he is capable of and should be engaging in. His foster parents should continue to demand *gradual* increments in responsive behavior. For instance, he would not be expected right away to put on his coat and button it, but he might be able to help by extending his arms or even slipping his arms into the sleeves as a first step.
2. R.'s verbal behavior is the outstanding area in which extensive professional help is needed. His communicative level is significantly below his general level of development. One-to-one contact with a professional speech therapist on an almost daily basis seems badly needed to try to stimulate and shape verbal behaviors. Short attention span could also be dealt with in that context. R.'s foster parents seem very open to professional direction and could greatly assist a speech therapy program by employing speech-eliciting techniques at home under the direction of R.'s speech therapist. (However, after his length of time in observation, we are not at all optimistic that intensive speech therapy will significantly alter the outcome.)

In spite of the poor prognosis, it is important that R. now has permanent parents in a stable home. These parents have been in-

cluded in R.'s evaluation each step of the way. They are fully aware
of the child's developmental problems. Although they maintain
considerable optimism, we have tried to dispel unrealistic expectations that could produce serious family stress in the future.

To some readers, R.'s case may seem extreme and unusual.
However, children with similar clinical pictures are referred
for psychiatric evaluation with considerable frequency. Often,
these children have been previously diagnosed as suffering Infantile Autism, Severe Mental Retardation, or both. The evidence of serial examinations of R. indicates that either diagnosis
alone may be misleading. These particular diagnostic labels can
instill an attitude of profound pessimism. Therefore, a definitive diagnostic label must be deferred unless the clinical findings are so obvious and conclusive that the clinician is left no
alternative. The goals in such cases as R. T.'s are to help the
guardians sustain attitudes of conservative optimism, meet
problems only as they arise, and institute remedial procedures
only when the child appears ready to benefit from them. Parents
usually need help in treading the narrow line between over-
protected infantilization and excessive pressure for achievement, both of which can impede the child's developmental
progress.

All but one of the cases presented (K. C.) showed rather profound disturbances in one or more areas of development. There
are many less severe psychiatric problems that occur in preschool children such as behavior problems, separation or other
anxiety disorders, withdrawal behavior, feeding problems, eating disorders, and sleep and bedtime and toilet training problems. Many times these symptoms are transient or are handled
by counseling of the parents by the primary care physician.
However, if these symptoms persist longer than a few weeks,
a complete psychiatric evaluation including a careful assessment of the psychologic state of the parents and family is indicated.

Empirically we have found that if the preschool child's overall developmental level is within the normal range the presenting symptoms are usually a reflection of some stress within
the family or a pathologic family interaction pattern. It is the
clinician's task to assess carefully the family as a whole as well
as each individual member, looking for possible pressures
and/or causes. A death in the family, chronic illness, especially
in the index child, and marital discord are common precipi-

tating stressors. Sometimes the child rearing practices are unwittingly precipitating or reinforcing undesirable behaviors or anxieties. If one or both parents suffer depression, psychosis, alcoholism or chronic neurosis an adverse effect on the child will usually occur. Occasionally, the full family evaluation is all that is needed in that the parents can correct the family stress once it has been made obvious. However, in many cases they need intensive and extensive family therapy, including individual psychopharmacologic therapy for one or more family members. Multiple therapists may become involved. Our clinic is a tertiary care facility. Therefore, in preschool children we seldom see psychiatric disorders that spontaneously remit. Some children may "outgrow" their problems, but we do not have the pleasure of seeing them.

SUMMARY

The examination of preschool children, especially if they have limited speech development, is quite difficult. These children must be examined within a developmental frame of reference rather than from the standpoint of differentiating specific mental disorders. The examiner must try to estimate the child's social age, verbal age, adaptive age and motor age.

Mental disturbances in preschool children are most clearly manifested by deviations in development, and parents are usually worried about the possibility of mental retardation and future inability to learn in school. Both emotional stress and biologic factors can interfere with early development. The differentiation of these two alternative causations can be extremely difficult. In fact, many times biologic and social factors are simultaneously interacting to produce the clinical manifestations of developmental impairment. Pinpointing the exact etiology and prognosticating can often be virtually impossible. The child's developmental level and rate must be studied by serial examinations. The clinician must assist the parents in correcting any pathogen that is rectifiable and in presenting properly timed remedial measures.

The technical problems of communicating with and relating to preschool children are discussed. Five cases are briefly presented to illustrate some of the variety of complex problems afflicting preschool children. The painstaking process needed for identifying developmental deviations and sorting their biologic, psychologic and social components is evident in the clinical examples.

Space limitations and copyright laws make it impossible to produce a complete, definitive course on early child developmental testing in this book. The clinician must have a solid background knowledge of child development if he intends to work with preschool children. Although it is unlikely that the busy physician will perform developmental testing himself, he must understand the basic principles underlying the 14 standardized preschool tests listed in the text of this chapter. In addition, we offer a "bare bones" list of references and suggested reading.[2,5,9–12]

In gaining proficiency with very small children, there is no substitute for experience and practice under supervision. Assignments to nursery schools, child development centers and well-baby clinics provide invaluable learning opportunities.

Treatment of preschool children with psychiatric disorders is sometimes relatively easy but can be long, arduous and full of tedium with an uncertain outcome. It must involve the family and often requires multiple therapists and a variety of kinds of therapy. As each month and year goes by without the child's progressing toward a modicum of normalcy or the family's adjusting to some form of chronic disability in the child, the prognosis for an extrainstitutional adjustment becomes more grim.

REFERENCES

1. American Psychiatric Association: *Diagnostic and Statistical Manual of Mental Disorders (DSM-III),* 3rd Ed. Washington, D.C., 1980, pp. 36–41 and 86–92.
2. DeMyer, M.K.: *Parents and Children in Autism.* Washington, D.C., V.H. Winston & Sons, 1979.
3. DeMyer, M.K., Barton, S., and Norton, J.A.: A comparison of adaptive, verbal and motor profiles of psychotic and non-psychotic subnormal children. J. Autism Child. Schizophr., 2:359, 1972.
4. DeMyer, M.K., Norton, J.A., and Barton, S.: Social and Adaptive Behaviors of Autistic Children as Measured in a Structured Psychiatric Interview, in *Infantile Autism,* Churchill, D., Alpern, G. and DeMyer, M.K. (Eds.). Springfield, Ill., Charles C Thomas, 1971.
5. Frankenburg, W.K., and Dodds, J.B.: *Denver Developmental Screening Test.* Denver, LADOCA Project and Publishing Foundation, 1969.
6. Freud, A.: *Normality and Pathology in Childhood: Assessments of Development.* New York, International Universities Profess., 1966.
7. Gesell, A., and Ilg, F.L.: *Infant and Child in the Culture of Today.* New York, Harper and Brothers, 1943.
8. Gesell, A., Ilg, F.L., and Ames, L.B.: *Infant and Child in the Culture of Today.* Revised Ed. New York, Harper and Row, 1974.

9. Meier, J.H.: Screening, assessment and intervention for young children at developmental risk, in *Intervention Strategies for High Risk Infants and Young Children,* Tjossem, T.D. (Ed.). Baltimore, University Park Press, 1976, pp. 251–387.
10. Province, S.: Developmental assessment, in *Ambulatory Pediatrics II* Green, M., and Haggerty, R.J. (Eds.). Philadelphia, W.B. Saunders Co., 1977, pp. 374–383.
11. Tarjan, G., et al. (Eds.): *The Physician and the Mental Health of the Child:* I. *Assessing Development and Treating Disorders Within a Family Context.* Chicago, American Medical Association, 1979.
12. *Ibid.: The Physician and the Mental Health of the Child:* II. *The Psychological Concomitants of Illness.* Chicago, American Medical Association, 1980.
13. Wilkins, T.J., and Campbell, J.L.: Psychosocial concerns in the paediatric burn unit. Burns, *7*:208–210. Printed in Great Britain, 1983.

7

NOSOLOGY AND DIAGNOSIS

Hunt, Wittson and Hunt[13] state that diagnosis is essentially a process of taxonomic categorization with prediction as its function. The accuracy of the prediction, of course, depends upon the accuracy of the diagnosis, which, in turn, implies as thorough knowledge as possible of the causation, the pathogenesis, and the natural course of the illness. An additional function of diagnosis is to allow professional communication.

DIAGNOSTIC CLASSIFICATION

According to the dictionary, the word *diagnosis* means "a process, the process of attempting to understand the patient."[22] It is also a short, scientific description (name) for taxonomic classification. Presumably, the more thorough the diagnostic process, the more accurate the taxonomic diagnosis and the more correct the treatment plan. Accurate diagnosis is always imperative for the patient and therapist. In addition, child psychiatry is still a relatively young medical specialty, and, thus, we are particularly concerned with improving our fundamental scientific bases and our communication with colleagues. A workable nomenclature is absolutely essential for scientific advancement.

Child psychiatry is living or repeating the growth and development of every other medical specialty. A scientific discipline begins with observations that are concrete enough to be seen and confirmed by others. Out of these findings, certain theoretical constructs are developed to help comprehend and make our observations useful. The theories are useful, but they do not constitute basic knowledge until they are shown to be reliable and valid.

RELIABILITY AND VALIDITY

At any given time in history, knowledge is a provisional state. It is achieved or accepted by a consensus that represents a compromise of the moment rather than a definitive achievement. Reliability is achieved through independent and simultaneous observation by more than one person. In medicine, we note empirically that certain signs and symptoms repeatedly cluster together, seeming to form a specific syndrome, disease or disorder that we name Syndrome "X." We consider this observation reliable (i.e., it truly does exist as a specific entity) if colleagues or trained observers can independently and simultaneously observe it. Syndrome "X" may exist, but is it valid? Does it bear a true, definite, strong relationship to what we think it is? Does it really measure or define a mental disorder from no mental disorder and one mental disorder from another? In matters of diagnosis (understanding), one can hope that our syndromes would also have validity for etiology, treatment and outcome. However, at this point in time, clinicians are so hopelessly divided regarding which etiologic and treatment theories to follow that we are indeed fortunate if we can achieve a diagnostic classification system at merely the descriptive level. In the past (before *DSM-III*), efforts to tie descriptive phenomena to specific etiologic theories have been confusing and disappointing.

The beginner clinician must understand the concepts of validity and reliability. He must know the usefulness and the limitations of diagnosis. Above all, he must conscientiously use diagnostic terms to convey understanding and avoid the danger of using scientific-sounding words as jargon that serves only to hide his ignorance. One must learn the diagnostic terms or language of one's discipline in order to communicate in a reliable way with one's colleagues. Having a diagnostic nomenclature is essential to provide a basis for research and administration. Arriving at a diagnostic name or label for the condition presented by the patient is also important for clinical practice, but it must be recognized as only an initial step in a comprehensive evaluation leading to the case formulation and a treatment plan. The diagnostic label should indicate what, descriptively, is wrong with your patient, but it cannot tell you why this syndrome or set of symptoms has occurred or what procedures or treatment approaches will most likely be helpful.

INTERNATIONAL STATISTICAL CLASSIFICATION OF DISEASES, INJURIES AND CAUSES OF DEATH (ICD)

About the beginning of this century, an International List of Causes of Death (ICD) was established in the medical world for statistical purposes. Through revisions at approximately 10-year intervals, the "list" was expanded to classify morbidity as well as mortality, with the new title "The International Statistical Classification of Disease, Injuries and Causes of Death" (still referred to as ICD). It was not until the fifth revision (1938) that a section on mental disorders was included, and reference to mental disorders specific for childhood and adolescence did not appear until 1977 *(ICD-9)*. Among the international community of psychiatrists there was considerable dissatisfaction with *ICD-6* (1948) and *ICD-7* (1955), and they were not widely used. As it became apparent that mental disorders constitute a serious international public health problem, the need for an acceptable classification of these disorders became most urgent. With support and action from the World Health Organization, there have been extensive revisions of the content and form of the mental disorders sections in *ICD-8* (1965) and *ICD-9* (1979).

DIAGNOSTIC AND STATISTICAL MANUAL OF MENTAL DISORDERS

In 1952, the American Psychiatric Association published its *Diagnostic and Statistical Manual of Mental Disorders (DSM-I)*.[2] This has had two revisions: *DSM-II* (1968) and *DSM-III* (1980).[4] In spite of considerable dissatisfaction and many shortcomings, *DSM-I* became rather widely used by psychiatrists practicing on the North American continent. The situation has developed that American physicians and hospitals use DSM classification and terms for mental disorders, and the ICD is used for the classification of all other diseases, injuries and causes of death. The committees of WHO and APA, who produced ICD and DSM respectively, have cooperated and made considerable effort to keep the two systems compatible. The DSM (1952) of the American Psychiatric Association was the first official manual of mental disorders to contain a glossary of descriptions of the diagnostic categories, and both ICD and DSM have had glossaries in their publications since 1960. Although considerable compatibility developed between the two systems, American psychiatrists remained concerned that the *ICD-9* classification and glossary were not suitable for use in the United States. Whether the remaining differences can be resolved to the extent that *DSM-IV* and *ICD-10* will be exactly the same in the near future remains to be seen.

DSM-I was considered totally unsatisfactory by most child psychiatrists, and it was ignored or used in a perfunctory manner by them, much to the consternation of statisticians, epidemiologists, hospital administrators, record librarians and public health officials, as well as the authors of *DSM-I*. In *DSM-II* (1968), particular attention was paid to disorders occurring in childhood that could not be accurately classified among the diagnostic categories traditionally used for illnesses occurring in adulthood. Even so, many child psychiatric clinicians remained uninterested. Those who attempted seriously to use *DSM-II* in working with children did so out of administrative necessity or a sense of duty, without enthusiasm. Child psychiatrists are few in number and nearly all of them are primarily clinicians rather than investigators or administrators. The overwhelming problems of child psychiatry were and are gross staff shortages; the complex tangle of etiologic factors and developmental phenomena; the great difficulty in clearly delineating child pathology, family or parental pathology and social pathology; plus the need for scientific validation or even rationale for our treatment methods, to name a few high priority issues. Intellectually, we welcomed *DSM-II* with the hope of bringing order out of chaos. Emotionally, we could not sense *DSM-II* as having any potential for contributing the answers and solutions we so urgently needed. The content and boundaries of *DSM-II* categories were not clearly enough defined. Diagnoses sometimes seemed based upon pure description, sometimes upon an etiologic theory, sometimes upon outcome and sometimes upon all of these factors. *DSM-II* did not make clear that children can suffer most of the syndromes seen in adults as well as those that appear first during childhood. The nature-nurture or organic-functional issues were compounded rather than clarified in *DSM-II*. No doubt, much of child psychiatry's dissatisfaction was due to an "expectation-reality discrepancy" (i.e., expecting more than was possible), compounded by the subspecialty's limited scientific data base and a zealous wish not to be hampered by limitations inherent in rigid, restricted nomenclature.

An example of child psychiatrists' themselves attempting to develop a classification for children's mental disorders is seen in the G.A.P. Report No. 62.[10] This work contains considerable symptom detail in order to convey as much as possible about the clinical condition and clearly to delineate one disorder from another. It attempts with only partial success to distinguish "Healthy Responses" and "Reactive Disorders" from more internalized and treatment-refractory conditions. It clearly shows that the major neuroses, psychoses and personality disorders do occur in childhood, and it gives due consideration to developmental phenomena. However, for many reasons, that G.A.P. report did not become widely used by the majority of child psychiatrists. In retrospect, it seems it was too difficult to learn to use and was not sufficiently superior to *DSM-I* and *II* to justify its adoption. About 1975, the American Psychiatric Association appointed a task force to prepare a third edition of the *Diagnostic and Statistical Manual of Mental Disorders*, better known as *DSM-III*, published in 1980.[4] Reactions from both child and adult psychiatrists have been quite favorable, and work has begun on an updated edition, *DSM (R)*, which is expected to be published in 1987.

Another valuable resource for the clinician is the classification in mental retardation produced by the American Association on Mental Deficiency.[9] They have kept their system compatible with *DSM-III* and ICD-9. The importance of not relying solely on a numerical IQ score for diagnosis is strongly emphasized. The following multiaxial coding system is used:

AXIS I: Intellectual functioning level
AXIS II: Etiology
AXIS III: Concurrent problems
AXIS IV: Psychosocial stressors

This system appears to be well suited for prognosticating and treatment planning for mental retardation and may be more uniquely tailored to the clinical issues of mental retardation than is the five-axial system of *DSM-III.*

The case material in this book has been classified whenever possible according to *DSM-III.* We urge all child psychiatric clinicians, both novice and seasoned, to read and learn to use *DSM-III* as quickly as possible. In fact, in the short period since its publication, this diagnostic manual has become so accepted and widely used that it would probably be impossible to pass the certifying examinations of the American Board of Psychiatry and Neurology, Inc., without a good working knowledge of *DSM-III.* It has become accepted in research as well as in clinical practice. *DSM-III's* prepublication field trials no doubt improved the eclecticism, making the nomenclature more acceptable and useful to a greater number of clinicians and investigators. A concerted effort has been made to restrict terms at the descriptive level, thus avoiding as much as possible vague, unproven or controversial postulates about etiology or prognosis. Although the Committee *(DSM-III)* did not reach a consensual definition of mental illness, they did reach a perhaps arbitrary agreement regarding what is *not* a mental disorder: "It is not a mental disorder if the disturbance is limited to a conflict between the individual and society." Although *DSM (R)* is expected to be even more useful, radical revisions of the nomenclature are not anticipated.

PRACTICAL USE OF *DSM-III*

From the viewpoint of many child psychiatrists, *DSM-III* is definitely an improvement over its predecessors. Rutter and Shaffer[20] have rather emphatically outlined what they consider serious oversights, ambiguities and unresolved issues in *DSM-III.* However, when comparing *DSM-III* with its predecessors *(DSM-I* and *II),* one is inclined to excuse the shortcomings or defer them to the future for correction by the DSM revision committee. *DSM-I* and *II* actually had little practical use in child psychiatry. We think this is not true for *DSM-III.* The disorders are clearly enough differentiated to make classification much less difficult and arbitrary. Children and adolescents are not set apart from adults as if they constituted a separate species. When symptoms occur that constitute a specific known disorder, they are so classified, whether the patient is an adult or child. The section on "Disorders Usually First Evident in Infancy, Childhood, or Adolescence" seems solidly based on current knowledge of early human development and the way it affects clinical pictures. For example, it has long been well known that a major psychosis can and does occur in children. Often, the clinical picture is quite different from a psychosis such as Schizophrenic Disorder seen in adulthood. Some of these children may have a juvenile version of a Schizophrenic Disorder. If this is true, these children's symptom clusters will increasingly resemble a Schizophrenic Disorder as the patients grow older.

Some of these children's symptoms may go into remission or remain but never clearly fit the category of Schizophrenic Disorders. When first seen in childhood, it is impossible to predict what direction the disturbance will take. It is much more accurate to have a category into which a child's symptoms fit at the time he is examined. The problem of trying to predict a future symptom picture then becomes unnecessary and irrelevant. We are only beginning to collect data showing which, if any, symptom clusters of childhood may bear a significant relationship to the various disorders seen among adults. For example, Attention Deficit Disorder and Conduct Disorder during prepuberty seem to be predisposing factors for adult Antisocial Personality Disorder. This is borne out by studies of the past histories of adults. Yet, we cannot predict anterospectively the future of children with these diagnoses. It may be that a specific childhood disorder is not predictive of anything, but some associated more subtle variables could be the significant predictive factors.

The manual instructs the clinician to consult first the section on "Disorders Usually First Evident in Infancy, Childhood, or Adolescence" when diagnosing someone who is not yet an adult. This may be confusing and seemingly contradictory. The body of the manual clearly indicates that the disorders in this section are *usually* "first evident" in infancy, childhood or adolescence. The age at which the person is examined is not an especially strong determinant of diagnosis. The age of *onset* of symptoms may be crucial for diagnosis. It is important for the clinician to remember that a child of 8 years may suffer "Conversion Disorder #300.81" and an adult, age 32, may be suffering "Childhood Onset Pervasive Developmental Disorder #299.9X." This is a significant issue. There has been a general tendency for those psychiatrists primarily working with children to ignore the nomenclature applied to adult patients and those working with adult patients to act as if the conditions that first appear in childhood are irrelevant. This schism is inaccurate and certainly counterproductive for the scientific advancement of psychiatry.

The multiaxial evaluation of *DSM-III* is very valuable. It clearly acknowledges that one diagnosis seldom, if ever, describes or accounts for all of the symptoms. It permits and ensures the inclusion of information that may be valuable, or even imperative, for treatment planning and prognosticating.

The clinician is not forced to choose between two or three diagnoses that are not mutually exclusive. For example:

"Phobic Neurosis" (DSM-II #300.2) in a child whose presenting complaint is "school refusal" tells you something about a child. The clinician might add, if appropriate, "in a child who is free of any other mental or physical disorder" or "in a child who also suffers mental retardation and Wilson's Disease."

With *DSM-III,* these two children would be classified as follows:

The child with no concomitant or complicating disorders would have the following diagnosis:

> Axis I: 309.21 Separation Anxiety Disorder
> Axis II: V71.09 No diagnosis on Axis II
> Axis III: None or no physical illness

The other child would have the following diagnosis:

> Axis I: 309.21 Separation Anxiety Disorder
>   317.0(X) Mild mental retardation
> Axis II: V71.09 No diagnosis on Axis II
> Axis III: Wilson's Disease (a hepatolenticular degeneration often
>   accompanied by mental retardation)

Since *DSM-III* came into use, we have insisted that our staff and students complete Axes IV and V even though hospital statisticians, administrators and third-party payors are only interested in Axes I, II and III. Axes IV and V have considerable relevance for prognostication and treatment planning. In general, the more severe a stressor has been and the higher the level of premorbid adjustment was, the better the prognosis. These two axes also should point out psychosocial stressors and adjustment problems that the therapist should especially keep in mind. This is true if there is a brief narrative description of the item(s) that led the evaluator to give that specific rating for that particular patient. Simple numerical ratings such as "Stress: #4, Moderate" or "Adjustment level: #4, Fair," are of much less value. Although the items on Axes IV and V are probably valid by virtue of their own definitions the actual numerical assignments are of necessity "judgment calls" of questionable reliability. Special attention to Axes IV and V ratings during staff conferences would probably increase their reliability among staff as well as between staff and students.

FAMILY DIAGNOSIS

Unfortunately, *DSM-III* does not attempt to classify family pathology, a subject increasingly being recognized as extremely important clinically. This intentional omission by the committee seems wise at this time. There are so few truly scientific data about families and such wide diversity among the theoretical schools of thought that a sound nomenclature and classification system for family pathology seems almost hopeless. In another 10 years or so a general consensus about a rational description and ordering for family pathology may be possible. Tseng and McDermott have offered a family classification proposal that is intriguing and may have some promise.[21] Also the classifications offered and reviewed by Beavers[5] seem to have considerable empirical logic. It may take many years for any family diagnostic classification system to demonstrate sufficient validity and reliability and ease of use that the majority of clinicians commonly employ it in their everyday practice. Only then is it likely that a diagnostic classification for family pathology will be included in a future APA diagnostic and statistical manual. Since family therapy is gaining rapidly as an appropriate and important form of treatment we need some method of succinctly designating what we are treating.

RELATING *DSM-III* DIAGNOSES TO SPECIFIC THERAPIES

Consideration has been given to classifying various treatment modalities relating specific treatments to the various conditions listed in *DSM-III.* Such a venture seems premature, grandiose and presumptuous. The idea completely ignores the lack of scientifically validated knowledge about treatment and outcome. Don Quixote may have been humanistic, admirable and lovable, but he is hardly a model to emulate completely. A "cookbook" for psychiatric practice carries the risk of arresting scientific advancement for decades. We must humbly accept the fact that the other, much older medical subspecialties have not been able to produce a "diagnostic-treatment" manual either. If clinicians of differing theoretical schools consistently use the same nomenclature for descriptive diagnoses, research toward finding the most effective treatments for different disorders can at least begin. The multiaxial system provides a rather broad view of all of the patient's problems. Planning treatment with due consideration for all of these variables and their interdigitations requires clinical judgment that cannot be reduced to a simple classification format.

DIAGNOSTIC CLASSIFICATIONS AND FORMULATIONS

In spite of its limitations for treatment planning, *DSM-III* is a giant step forward for child psychiatry. Ideally, our nomenclature should designate specific types of disorders (symptom complexes), the manner of their development (pathogenesis), their separate causes and their prognoses. Rutter[19] stresses that a diagnostic classification should convey important and relevant information about the patient, but that one should not expect it to say all that is relevant or important. Many clinicians believe that we should use the terms *diagnostic classification* and *diagnostic formulation* separately to avoid compounding our confusion about psychopathology.

The purpose of the *DSM-III* scientific nomenclature or categorization is to order our knowledge of childhood psychopathology in such a way that it can be succinctly and accurately communicated to others. The purpose of a "diagnostic formulation" is to provide the basis for a rational treatment approach for one specific child. Classification must be based upon reproducible facts and not upon speculative concepts. Such scientific rigidity is neither possible nor particularly desirable in a diagnostic formulation. The nomenclature is for the classification of disorders, not of children. A diagnostic formulation is for the planning of treatment for a specific child, not for the ordering of childhood disorders.

As progress is made, we would expect the differences between the diagnostic classification of a child's illness and the diagnostic formulation to become fewer. We would never expect the two concepts to be so identical, however, that we cease treating children with emotional problems and treat only an emotional disorder that happens to have afflicted a child. Classification involves study of the common characteristics of large groups of subjects, whereas a diagnostic formulation involves the clinical study, in depth, of the uniqueness of an individual patient.

The members of the various committees who worked so diligently to produce *DSM-III* can take pride in the fact that no longer is diagnostic classification either ignored or deprecated. We may be on the threshold of some very important scientific discoveries now that psychiatrists have reached some consensus on what it is that we want to study and/or treat. In spite of our theoretical differences, we can talk with each other about our patients now. Knowledge of the problems of nomenclature seems essential to the understanding of patients and to the meaningful integration of the mental status examination into the diagnostic formulation.

ETIOLOGY AND TREATMENT ARE NOT SELF-EVIDENT FROM A DIAGNOSTIC LABEL

Even though *DSM-III* categories are in a developmental context, descriptive classification of mental disorders is especially difficult in child psychiatry because the patient is still a growing, developing organism. The psychic structure remains in a fluid state. Age may color or even be a major determinant in the symptom picture or in the vulnerability to stress.

Etiology is also difficult to incorporate in any classification system. Behavior and thinking are multidetermined. Therefore, in pathologic states, multiple causation is the rule, and a single cause directly related to a specific condition is rare or nonexistent. Different etiologic factors may cause similar symptom pictures; varying symptom complexes may be caused by the same etiologic agents. For example, children with demonstrable brain damage may show thinking and behavior disturbances similar to those in youngsters with no evidence of central nervous system disorder. The structural and physiologic interrelationships of the central nervous system have rendered attempts to correlate certain behavior deviations with localized lesions fruitless even with the exciting discoveries in the area of neurohormones.

When central nervous system abnormalities can be demonstrated, the direct relation of the organic disturbance to specific psychic or behavioral symptoms is often questionable. Children with brain damage frequently show disturbed interpersonal and intrafamily relationships. The question of which is primary and which is secondary may rest more with the theoretical biases of the investigator than with the objective facts. The problem of determining primary cause(s) may seem merely to be an academic exercise for the psychiatrist. Nevertheless, his conclusions about the relation of pathologic findings to the clinical problems are immediately crucial to treatment planning.

Most youngsters seen in office practice or in child guidance clinics bear no evidence of central nervous system malfunctioning. Careful history taking produces ample evidence of disturbed or traumatic relationships and events within the past and present environments to support the thesis of a functional origin, but types of interpersonal dysfunctions and their relation to specific clinical symptoms are not definitely established. In general, the severity of the effect of psychologic trauma is inversely proportional to the age of the child and directly proportional to the duration of the stress, yet genetic, constitutional, sociologic and other variables prevent this latter statement from becoming more than a generalization.

Psychoanalytic theories have been helpful in clarifying some of these relations between events and behavior. Within the analytic context, the relation of ego functioning to past and present relationships and events has become clinically more understandable. Menninger et al.[18] have proposed that many forms of behavior that are termed "symptoms" may be the organism's attempts at restitution or the maintenance of psychologic homeostasis in the face of either internal or external stresses. Some patients may have failed to develop in certain ways. Others appear to have regressed to more immature mechanisms for coping with either organic or psychic assaults. Such theoretical constructs are extremely useful in planning psychologic therapy or corrective procedures. Nevertheless, the difficulty in establishing direct cause-and-effect relations between events and behavior and the high degree of variability from individual to individual make these constructs extremely difficult to integrate into any system of diagnostic classification. Clinical observation has confirmed that disturbed behavior and many psychic symptoms are reminiscent of, or even almost identical with, earlier (younger) modes of reacting. In dealing with children, however, the matter of age-appropriateness for various behaviors is subject to clinical judgment and much debate.

Anna Freud[7] describes an interesting obstacle to any definitive etiologic classification of mental disorders in children. She points out that temporary ego regressions are a part of normal child development. They may be a reaction to everyday stresses of tiredness, anxiety of separation or physical illness. In addition, the growth process itself broadens the child's reality awareness and exposes him to many painful and anxiety-provoking aspects of life. Freud's thesis is a confirmation of the fact that no child's development progresses along a steady linear course, but that children take two steps forward and one step backward in their maturation. Such regressions appear to be beneficial if they are temporary and spontaneously reversible. However, prolongation of regression may result in disturbances of relationships and become a pathogenic agent in itself. The situation is further complicated by the difficulty in differentiating temporary from more permanent regressions and accurately predicting a spontaneous return to previous levels of adjustment. Parents give recognition to this phenomenon when they ask, "Is he emotionally ill or is he just going through a stage?"

THE DIAGNOSTIC FORMULATION

Difficult though it may be to relate diagnostic classification to specific treatment, the clinician need not despair of helping his patient. He can develop a diagnostic formulation and rational treatment plan based upon knowledge of the individual patient and the accumulated body of theory and facts about childhood emotional disorders. Our concept of diagnostic formulation is similar to what Menninger[17] has termed *diagnostic synthesis,* and the "Dynamic Genetic Formulation" outline in the Appendix of G.A.P. Report No. 62.[11] Detailed comprehension of the multiple determinants of individual personality functioning is vital to intelligent clinical management.

The clinician must be familiar with the literature and have some clinical psychiatric experience in order to participate in either diagnostic or therapeutic work with children. Comprehension of the diagnostic formulation requires some understanding of sociomedical history taking and the multidisciplinary team approach that have been the *modus operandi* of clinical child psychiatry for the past 40 to 50 years. The beginner is urged to read Report No. 38 of the Group for the Advancement of Psychiatry (G.A.P.)[10] for a brief review of long-accepted practices in child guidance clinics. In Chapter 9, this author will also review a case history outline and case material to demonstrate the integration of data about the physical, emotional and social aspects of the past and present life of the child into a formulation and treatment plan.

The diagnostic formulation and treatment plan contain the answers, so far as these are possible, to eight implicit questions:
1. How sick or impaired is this child?
2. In what areas of his functioning is the impairment manifested and in what areas does he function well? (See Outline for Mental Status Examination of a Child, Chapter 4.)
3. Is there any past or present evidence that the central nervous system is not functionally intact?
4. What psychosocial factors in his past life have probably contributed to the problem?
5. Which psychosocial factors in his current life continue to contribute to his problem or are likely to be an impediment to recovery?
6. Which of the factors in questions 2, 3, 4 and 5 is it imperative to change in order for improvement to occur?
7. Which factors in questions 2, 3, 4 and 5 would the clinician desire to change for the general well-being of the child, although perhaps not essential for change in the child's presenting problems?
8. What methods, if any, can be used to effect the desired changes noted in questions 6 and 7?

All these questions are related to three basic issues: in what manner is this child's functioning impaired, why is this so, and what can be done about it? These questions do not separate easily. This difficulty in separating cause and effect may explain why some centers tend to treat all children with a "shotgun" therapeutic approach, or why the work of other centers seems to confirm and reinforce preconceived theories about the major causes and most effective treatment approaches to most childhood emotional problems. The foregoing eight-item breakdown in the diagnostic formulation considers the fact that there are usually multiple impairments and multiple causes. Empirically, prognosis seems to have a direct quantitative relation to questions 1 through 5. Although qualitative factors also play a role in prognosis, the greater the number of disturbed ego functions (question 2) and the greater the number of apparent contributing causes (questions 3, 4 and 5), the worse the outlook seems to be.

In our experience, the most severely disabling illnesses seen in childhood, the pervasive developmental disorders, show moderate to severe deviations in all or nearly all the items listed in the mental status examination. The prognosis is uniformly guarded for all of these children. It is commonly assumed that psychotic children with demonstrable central nervous system pathology have an even worse prognosis than those with no organic impairment. Nevertheless, a child with a neurologic impairment living in an intact family may have a considerably better chance of at least social recovery than a neurologically nonimpaired child living in a severely disturbed psychosocial environment. Actually, a child with both impairment of brain functioning and a problematic situation in his environment may have the least chance of all for attaining reasonably normal adjustment levels.

A low number and mild degree of ego deviations (question 2) do not necessarily indicate that the child will spontaneously improve or be treated easily. A child with severe anxiety who displays many neurotic defense mechanisms may respond well to outpatient psychotherapy, provided he has a reasonably intact superego, demonstrates the capacity for meaningful interpersonal relations (see question 2), and has family members who are relatively free of unchangeable neurotic interaction patterns that perpetuate his problems (see question 5). Major differences in the answers to questions 2 and 5 for a particular child could alter the situation to the extent that outpatient psychotherapy alone would not be sufficient treatment.

The number of possible answers to each of the foregoing eight questions and the number of possible combinations of answers make it impractical to outline absolute rules for treatment programming or prognostication in every conceivable type of case. Diagnosis and treatment depend upon clinical experience and judgment. The information gathered from the psychiatrist's examination, supplemented by social history and psychologic data, should provide answers to the first four questions. The detailed social history and evaluation of the parents supply answers to questions 5 and 6. On the basis of the total information, treatment planning and prognosis are formulated. In some of the case illustrations in the preceding chapters, we have outlined what seemed to us appropriate treatment plans, and we will give more examples in the chapters that follow.

SUMMARY

Diagnostic classification of childhood mental disorders and the diagnostic formulation of a particular child's disability are two somewhat overlapping tasks that have distinctly different objectives. Classification serves to organize the accumulated body of knowledge of the psychopathology of childhood for the clinician and the scientific investigator. Formulation of a specific child's disability serves as a rational basis for designing a treatment plan for that child. We must strive for knowledge that will make classification and diagnostic formulations similar and complementary to each other. It is neither possible nor desirable at this time, however, to make these two clinical, scientific functions identical in process or aim.

An overview and critique of the American Psychiatric Association's efforts to develop a classificatory nomenclature (*DSM-I, II* and *III*)[2–4] has been presented. Now, more than 30 years later *[DSM-I* (1952) to *DSM-III* (1980)]*, we believe the nomenclature for mental disorders occurring in children is clear and useful enough that child psychiatrists can use it in practice and teach it to their students.

A diagnostic formulation outline consisting of eight questions has been offered. Several of these questions can be answered only by history and by examination of significant elements of the child's environment. History taking,[10,12] family dynamics,[1,23] psychologic testing,[8,14] and child neurology[6,15,16] are reviewed elsewhere in the literature. This material was not reviewed in the text but is offered as supplemental reading.

The first six chapters of this text discussed the examination of the family's interaction and the child's mental status examination. In the next chapter, we will briefly review history taking and demonstrate ways the history, psychologic testing, and mental status examination may be integrated into a complete case study and diagnostic formulation leading to a treatment plan.

REFERENCES

1. Ackerman, W.W.: *Psychodynamics of Family Life.* New York, Basic Books, 1958.
2. American Psychiatric Association: *Diagnostic and Statistical Manual of Mental Disorders (DSM-I).* Washington, D.C., 1952.
3. ———: *Diagnostic and Statistical Manual of Mental Disorders (DSM-II),* 2d. Ed. Washington, D.C., 1968.
4. ———: *Diagnostic and Statistical Manual of Mental Disorders (DSM-III),* 3d Ed. Washington, D.C., 1980.
5. Beavers, W.R. and Voeller, M.N.: Family models: Comparing and contrast-

ing the Olson circumplex model with the Beavers systems model. Fam. Proc., *27*:85–98, 1983.

6. Dodge, P.R.: Neurologic history and examination, in *Pediatric Neurology*, Farmer, T.W. (Ed.). New York, Harper & Row, 1964.

7. Freud, A.: Regression as a principle in mental development. Bull. Menninger Clin., *27*:126, 1963.

8. Goodenough, F.L.: *Measurement of Intelligence by Drawings*. World Book Co., 1926.

9. Grossman, H.J. (Ed.): *Classification in Mental Retardation*. American Association on Mental Deficiency, 8th Ed., Washington, D.C., 1983.

10. Group for the Advancement of Psychiatry: *The Diagnostic Process in Child Psychiatry, Report No. 38*. New York, 1957.

11. ———: *Psychopathological Disorders in Childhood; Theoretical Considerations and a Proposed Classification, Report No. 62*. New York, 1966.

12. Hamilton, G.: *Psychotherapy in Child Guidance*. New York, Basic Books, 1947.

13. Hunt, W.A., Wittson, C.L. and Hunt, E.B.: A theoretical and practical analysis of the diagnostic process, in *American Psychopathological Association Proceedings, 41*:55. New York, Grune & Stratton, 1953.

14. Klopfer, B. (Ed.): *Developments in Rorschach Technique*. New York, Grune & Stratton, 1963.

15. Koppitz, E.: *The Bender-Gestalt Test for Young Children*. New York, Grune & Stratton, 1963.

16. Mayo Clinic: *Clinical Examination in Neurology*, 2d. Ed. Philadelphia, W.B. Saunders Co., 1963.

17. Menninger, K.: *A Manual for Psychiatric Case Study*, 2d. Ed. New York, Grune & Stratton, 1962.

18. Menninger, K., Mayman, M. and Pruyser, P.: *The Vital Balance*. New York, Viking Press, 1963.

19. Rutter, M.: Classification and categorization in child psychiatry. J. Child Psychol. Psychiatry, *6*:71, 1965.

20. Rutter, M. and Shaffer, D.: DSM-III: A step forward or back in terms of the classification of child psychiatric disorders? J. Amer. Acad. Child Psychiatry, *15*:15, 1976.

21. Tseng, W.S. et al.: Family diagnosis and classification. J. Amer. Acad. Child Psychiatry, *15*:15, 1976.

22. *Webster's New World Dictionary of the American Language*, 2d. College Ed., Guralnik, D.B. (Ed.-in-Chief). Cleveland and New York, William Collins and World Publishing Co., Inc., 1976, p. 388.

23. Zuk, G. and Rubenstein, D.: A review of concepts in the study and treatment of families of schizophrenics, in *Intensive Family Therapy*, Boszormenyi-Nagy, I. and Framo, J.L. (Eds.). New York, Harper & Row, 1965, pp. 1–32.

8

INTERVIEWING THE PARENTS

Obtaining the history of the patient has been an accepted practice for so long that any questions about it or review of its content may seem to be unnecessary. Even so, the history of the child psychiatric patient has such special significance that it deserves separate consideration.

The direct psychiatric examination of the child has been discussed in detail first in this monograph to underscore its importance. However, as stated in earlier sections, certain facts essential for diagnosis and treatment planning can be obtained only from the parents. These particulars, essentially unknown to the child, are his early development, past physical and psychologic stresses, comparison of his social-developmental level with that of his age group, characteristics of the parental relationship, and an objective assessment of the emotional well-being of each parent.

In addition, in the past 15 to 20 years we have become aware of the importance of understanding the relative health or pathology of the whole family and the interactions of the family subsystems (see Chapter 2).

TWO DISPARATE ATTITUDES

The approach to the parents can be considered from two extreme but inaccurate points of view. One position is that the parents are without a doubt the direct cause of the child's symptoms. Any information to the contrary arises merely from parental resistance to accepting the blame and taking corrective measures. The opposite stance is that parents have unjustifiably been made scapegoats by child development theorists. In this view, children's symptoms are seen as the result of some quirk of fate, "bad seed," or elusive organic central nervous system impairment. Hence, parents are interviewed for the sole purpose of obtaining an "objective" history of the child's symptoms and development. Those with this latter attitude toward parents consider the emotional interplay within the family irrelevant. Some students readily sympathize with cooperative, poised, interested parents who share the student's own value system. However, they make whipping boys of parents who are inarticulate or whose views on race, religion, politics, sex, child rearing, and other sociocultural phenomena are different from the interviewer's.

Behavioral scientists and serious students of human behavior strive for objectivity and take pride in any success they achieve in freeing themselves of biases. Even so, it is often impossible to know whether certain parental attitudes or practices are truly pathogenic or are merely called deviant because they are distasteful or incomprehensible to the investigator. Sears et al.[17] document the great variety of childhood experiences evident among American children of a similar sociocultural economic class and the tremendous task of relating these experiences to specific aspects of each child's personality. Clinical experience, research, and common sense tell us that all parents influence the behavior and development of their child in an infinite number of ways. Even so, we must await much more extensive basic research in the behavior sciences before we can completely understand the complicated interplay between the environmental experiences and the genetic-constitutional endowment of the child that underlie each symptom complex.

At least current knowledge and practices have made the old game of either condemning or exonerating parents as outdated as the controversy of organic versus functional etiology. In some cases, parental attitudes and behavior are highly relevant to the child's problems. In other cases, circumstances of fate or the child's native personality endowment are more important. In still other situations, a complicated admixture of the child's temperament and his life experiences is the only logical explanation for his symptom picture or his developmental direction.[6]

To achieve an accurate and useful diagnostic formulation, the clinician must maintain the same sympathetic, inquisitive approach to the parents that he has toward the child. By conscientiously trying to obtain an impression of both the assets and liabilities of each parent's personality and their relationship with each other and with their child, the interviewer should be able to prevent his own value judgments from distorting the interview process.

Premature efforts to differentiate "normal" and "pathologic" parental behavior should be avoided. Such "good" and "bad" judgments on isolated bits of behavior are likely to reflect the clinician's feelings about his own upbringing and have only incidental relevance to the problems presented by the patient. For many years, investigators attempted to relate specific parental behaviors such as breast- or bottle-feeding, types of discipline, and time and methods of toilet training to personality traits or later behavioral symptoms in the child. No such specific correlations have ever been convincingly demonstrated between parental actions and child behaviors. Research then turned from what parents do to the study of what parents think and feel (attitudes). Zuckerman,[21,22] Mark,[11] Shoben,[18] Becker[1] and others have attempted to use consciously stated parental attitudes to differentiate parents of normal children from parents of maladjusted children without success. Gildea et al.[7] found little relationship between specific parental attitudes and adjustment in a group of schoolchildren. However, they did feel that there were significant relationships between "patterns of attitude combinations and adjustment." The interviewer needs to know each parent's attitude and the affective experiences associated with the pregnancy and birth. The times and ways the child was fed, trained, disciplined, loved, and taught about property rights, sex, and so on, are all important. However, it is the total shape or arrangement of the parent-child and family interactions that is important to his development. Isolated events that the parents can describe or that can be observed, together with understanding of the parents' strengths and weaknesses, must be woven into patterns that portray the daily emotional life of the child.

Currently, much attention is being directed toward family interaction patterns as well as individual parental pathology. Using the MMPI, McAdoo and Connolly[13] and McAdoo[12] studied adults who were parents of child guidance clinic patients and adult psychiatric outpatients who were also parents of young children. Using Goldberg's classification, they found that significantly more mothers and fathers of the child guidance sample were classified as normal than the corresponding parents who were themselves outpatients. Although many investigators have found that parents of children with psychiatric problems have a higher number of psychiatric problems than parents of problem-free children, McAdoo's study demonstrated that the MMPI profiles of child guidance parents more closely resemble those of parents of children without emotional disorder than those of adult outpatients who are also parents. A definite relation of the elevated parental MMPI profile to the children's problems could not be shown. In any event, parental psychopathology is important to treatment planning, whether or not it bears an etiologic relationship to the child's disorder. Sometimes parental psychopathology may reinforce the child's symptoms with secondary gain or interfere with the parent's full cooperation in treatment.

Tseng and McDermott[20] have proposed a triaxial system for classifying functions and dysfunctions associated with the family. A valid and reliable method of identifying the functions and dysfunctions within the family would be extremely valuable for treatment planning and could lead to more refined research into cause and effect relationships.

On the basis of their longitudinal study of 136 children for more than 10 years, Chess et al.[2] also conclude that "parent-child interaction should be analyzed not only for parental influences on the child but just as much for the influence of the child's individual characteristics on the parent." For more than 30 years, many investigators[3–5,14–16] have clearly described significant psychopathology and social pathology often seen in parents and families of symptomatic children. Although such studies have been extremely useful to clinicians, exact cause-effect phenomena remain somewhat elusive. One remains at a loss to explain the asymptomatic children in these families, and it is often impossible to be certain whether it is the parents' pathology or the child's that is the primary factor in the clinical picture.

INTERVIEWING VERSUS HISTORY TAKING

I have called this chapter "Interviewing the Parents" in preference to "History Taking" because of the broader implication of the term *interview*. It is essential to have a historical account of the child's presenting problems, the course of symptoms, his current overall adjustment, and his past physical and psychologic development from conception to the present time. However, we also need data about the past and present emotional climate of the home and an assessment of the physical and mental health of each parent. These data are not only important to etiology and diagnosis but should be highly influential in determining the choice of treatment and the prognosis. The natural dependency of the child makes the parent an essential party to his treatment as well as to his pathology.

Simmons[19] has reviewed methods for sociomedical-psychologic history taking in a pediatric outpatient clinic. The same principles apply to the history of a child with an identifiable emotional problem. A noncondemning, fact-gathering approach helps to lessen parental guardedness and defensiveness. To enhance the accuracy of the history and to obtain the maximum parental cooperation, the necessity of interviews with each parent by oneself or by a member of one's own staff cannot be overemphasized.

Helper[8] and Levitt[9] have found low agreement between children's self-evaluations and evaluations of them by their parents. Clinically, it is often evident that the parents have quite different ideas about their child and each other. It is, therefore, important to review the salient points of the history in a family group interview (see Chapter 2) and to see the parents together without the child as well as to interview each parent alone. When the child lives full- or part-time with both parents, direct interviews with each of them is necessary for an accurate history. The old practice of seeing only the mother and child has been discarded in favor of interviewing the mother-father-child triad or even including entire families in the diagnosis and treatment. The subtle interaction patterns that constitute family relationships cannot be comprehended without firsthand acquaintance with all of the principals.

An outline for recording the child's and the family's history follows. In addition, the examiner needs to know something of each parent's personal adjustment and reaction patterns within the family. It could be said that we need to have a mental status examination of each parent. However, a comparatively brief, personal sociomedical-psychologic history is probably more palatable to the parents and more accurately reflects current practices. Following is an abbreviated list of topics and questions to be discussed in the parent interviews. Of course, the parents should not be vigorously interrogated on each of these subjects. They should be permitted to tell their story spontaneously in their own manner. The interviewer should guide the discussion in order that the various topics are covered in whatever order the parents' comfort indicates.

OUTLINE FOR INTERVIEWING THE PARENTS

1. Child's history
   a. Parents' main concerns about the child (chief complaint or presenting problem)
   b. Course of symptoms and current adjustment
   c. Past developmental, medical, social, and psychologic history, including peer and school adjustments
   d. Child's relationships with siblings and each parent
   e. Events that motivated them to seek help now
2. Parents' marital history
3. Parents' personal history
   a. Parents' primary family, past and present
   b. School and vocational adjustment
   c. Social and avocational interests and activities
   d. Review of any specific medical or psychologic problems suffered by either parent
4. Other family problems (other children, previous marriages, grandparents, parents' siblings, neighbors, and so on)
5. Parents' opinions about possible causes, and a review of their feelings about various treatments that might be proposed

Child's History

Most parents are defensive about their child. The defensiveness and guardedness are enhanced if the parent is asked to tell what's "wrong" or what he "thinks" is wrong with the child. Words like *wrong, bad, problem,* and *trouble* are best avoided. An invitation to describe or tell about the child gives unspoken recognition of normal parental ambivalence and encourages the parent to state both his positive and negative views of the child's adjustment. Many parents very easily and spontaneously give a full history of the child with little prodding or direction from the interviewer. If parents seem to be at a loss for words or to be holding back information, questions regarding dates and circumstances of significant events or developmental milestones can help to get them started talking. As the parents relax, inquiry can then be made into emotionally charged symptoms or events if these facts are not spontaneously related.

Parents' knowledge of the child and family lies in three levels of their consciousness. First, there are facts and opinions that are in the foreconscious and that will be told readily to almost anyone. Second, there are certain points that are consciously withheld from the interviewer because of distrust, fear of embarrassment, or the parents' belief that they are not relevant to the examination. Finally, there is a wealth of valuable data that the parents have repressed or forgotten because of their emotional charge. If the interviewer-parent relationship promotes trust and is skillfully directed, parents voluntarily reveal more and more about themselves and the family. This process in turn stimulates associations and often releases repressed material. Frequently, parents themselves are surprised at the many forgotten but significant events that come to their minds as a result of the interviews. Of course, much important repressed material cannot be released during diagnosis but must await therapy when indicated.

If the preceding suggestions do not facilitate the parent's verbal productivity, it can be assumed that the cause of the reticence lies with some factor outside the immediate interviewer-parent relationship. Paucity of words may be merely a personality characteristic of the parent, and nothing can be done but record it as an observation. Frequently, though, defensiveness is caused by feelings of shame or anger or the circumstances surrounding the referral. Inquiry into the parent's concept of the child's or family's need for help should bring out these feelings. Often it is necessary to permit the parent to spend considerable time ventilating his anger about the referring individual or agency before he can give the child's history.

Mr. R. appeared impatient and irritable. He did not talk spontaneously. When asked to tell his reasons for bringing his son, Mike, for examination, he replied, "They say he has a school problem." In response to the query of what Mr. R. considered Mike's school problem to be, he said, "He (apparently meaning the teacher or principal) said Mike acted up in class, disturbed the other kids, and last week pushed a boy down the steps. I don't know what's wrong over at that school, but we don't have trouble like that around home. The schools today don't even try to have good discipline." The interviewer commented that the family must be pretty annoyed to have Mike sent for examination with false accusations. Mr. R. responded that the allegations may have been partially true but he resented Mike's being singled out. The school certainly had plenty of children whose behavior was worse. He then launched into a lengthy discussion of the school's discrimination against laboring-class families. There were plenty of rumors about the principal's being incompetent and possibly immoral. Many parents are ready to expose the fact that most of the teachers are unfit for their jobs. After considerable ventilation, Mr. R. stated that Mike had probably done those things, but "He is not a mental case." His mother couldn't handle him, but that was her fault. Mr. R. had repeatedly told her to crack down. She was always tired out and depressed. She babied the boy and then complained to him. "Mike is no mental case." He knows better. He never acted that way when the father was home. "I won't stand for it. The school and his mother ought to thrash him. I've told them to."

Having released much feeling, Mr. R. was then able to give other information about his child and family fairly easily.

Parents' Marital History

The marital relationship is a very private and sensitive topic that must be approached forthrightly but with tact and discretion. This subject might be introduced by a statement that many parents are surprised and embarrassed that we ask personal questions about their relationship with their marital partner. However, in the interest of helping us understand their child, we hope they will answer such questions to the best of their ability. Such a direct request for cooperation is reassuring to the parents and is seldom refused. Some discuss their associations with their spouses readily. Whether they do so easily or not, it is important to know the length of courtship, ages at the time of marriage, reactions of family to the marriage, type of family planning if any, and who has assumed the dominant role regarding money, decisions, child discipline, the sexual adjustment, and so forth. What was the reason for the marriage? This may be approached by inquiry into what attracted the parents to each other. The romantic idea of intense, irresistible love is probably responsible for much less than half the marriages. Frequently, marital discontent is due to unfulfilled fantasies about what the marriage should be, even though these wishes or hopes were never verbalized even to the self. Multiple marriages and separations for any reason must be inquired about. Often the diagnostic inquiry brings about the parent's first reflection on the child's reactions to such events. Direct questions about infidelity must be asked since such information is seldom volunteered.

Parents' Personal History and Attitudes toward Treatment

Individuals who can talk about the foregoing topics usually have little difficulty giving their own personal history. The simple explanation should be given that it will help in the understanding of the patient if we know something of each parent's primary family and upbringing. The interviewer cannot be satisfied with the statement that "My own childhood was normal" without knowing the informant's concept of normalcy. The culture and the early relationships and events that have influenced the mother's or father's attitudes and behavior about parenthood are important to know.

The novice may have some reluctance about exploring the parents' personal and family histories, feeling that time may be wasted obtaining irrelevant data and not being certain about what types of topics need exploration in depth. A few guiding principles may help.

First, if the appropriate questions are not asked, important information may be overlooked. It is known that genetic and/or familial factors are frequently quite relevant if one suspects a major psychosis, an affective disorder, alcoholism, mental retardation or an antisocial personality disorder. In such instances a mental health history of both parents, the grandparents and the parents' siblings must be determined. Quite frequently in cases of child abuse the parent(s) were also abused as children, and tactful inquiry must be made about this point.

Most parents try not to emulate their own parents in matters of child rearing blindly. Yet it is a fact that our basic and most influential lessons in this subject come from positive and negative experiences during our lives with our own parents. In cases of suspected parent-child relationship problems one needs a detailed account of the relationship of each parent to each of his own parents. Many good clues for treatment can be found in such information.

All children form some close identifications with their parents, particularly the parent of the same sex. One must ask both parents whether they had similar symptoms or problems as children. They may have forgotten or believed such information not to be important. Given time the parent will usually give the facts.

Timothy, age 4½ years, was brought to the child psychiatrist by his father for psychotherapy for his speech problem. The father was a professional person with several advanced academic degrees. He was certain that Tim's speech was due to chronic anxiety and that he needed psychotherapy or psychotropic medication or both.

Tim's speech was barely comprehensible. His voice had a nasal quality. In addition to a lisp, his articulation and enunciation were far from normal. The nasopharynx and hearing were normal. He did seem to be quite tense and anxious. The anxiety could have been a reaction to his problem in communicating rather than a cause of the speech difficulty.

The examiner noticed that the father's speech had some similar characteristics. There was the same deep nasal sound. He articulated slowly and carefully, but when he discussed an emotionally charged topic he was barely understandable. When inquiry was made about the similarity in the speech, the father seemed startled. It simply had not occurred to him that Timmy had the same problem as he. He had struggled with it all of his life. As a small child he had been shamed, ridiculed and punished for it, making the problem worse.

It was recommended that Tim have intensive speech therapy. We were not sure whether psychotherapy could help or were needed. The child was to be brought back at 6-month intervals for further assessment of the need for psychotherapy. Unfortunately, the family moved out of the state because of the father's work, and we do not have a completed follow-up. We do know that the child entered regular public kindergarten before the move.

Children's unconscious imitation of parents can be seen in their gestures, gait, speech, and even sometimes in a psychosomatic disorder.

Carolyn, age 10½ years, had had several hospital evaluations for her chronic abdominal pain without any physical causes being uncovered. Her pediatric intern in presenting the case described her as a bright, affable little girl who worried constantly about the possibility of having surgery. She was certain that she would have to have an operation on this admission. She even seemed to look forward to it. The intern was perplexed about why this child or any other would want surgery. He was asked how much surgery the mother had had. He didn't know and wondered whether that was important. He was instructed to get the history so that its importance could then be discussed. A short time later he reported, "The mother has had only eleven abdominal operations but the maternal grandmother has had thirty-three." Further discussion of the importance of the family history was unnecessary.

Specific treatment recommendations cannot be made until the study is completed. Nevertheless, some preliminary discussion of the family's reactions to various possible treatment plans have both therapeutic and prognostic value. Previous treatments and corrective procedures considered by the parents should be reviewed. The most frequent recommendations for child psychiatric problems are individual psychotherapy for one or more members of the family, group therapy, conjoint therapy, family group therapy, tutoring and remedial education, and environmental manipulations such as adjustments of school curriculum, change of schools, boarding school, residential treatment school, or hospital. In addition, one of the psychotropic medications may be included in the final recommendation.

The treatment possibilities most likely for the case at hand should be explained to the parents. Their response often reveals the degree to which they understand the child's symptoms and the degree to which they personally are able or willing to participate in treatment. In addition, pragmatic issues such as cost, frequency of visits, length of treatment, distance of home from the treatment center, and availability of community resources nearer their home all have a direct bearing on parental acceptance of the final recommendations and are significant for prognostication.

Levitt[10] postulated that expectation-reality discrepancy (ERD) is negatively related to favorable therapy outcome. He recommends education of the patient (and parent) about her/his role in treatment. Reduction of the difference between the patient's expectations of what therapy will be like and what really will occur can have a "catalytic effect" on treatment outcome. Simply stated, it seems reasonable that a good rational, intelligent grasp of various corrective procedures is essential for maximum parental cooperation. Hence, a systematic review of various forms of treatment is needed to give the parents some intellectual understanding of the various types of corrective procedures that may be recommended for their child.

SUMMARY

In this book we have emphasized the importance of directly interviewing the child patient, feeling that in the literature and in practice there has been too much reliance on the history as given by the parent and too little attention paid to careful examination of the child. However, we do not intend to minimize or overlook the importance of obtaining a careful history from the parents. This chapter has reviewed some general principles regarding parent interviews.

The clinician must avoid blaming the parent for all of the child's problems. On the other hand he should not overlook the fact that parental personalities and family events are relevant to the child's personality development. To obtain accurate historical data and to comprehend the subtle family interaction patterns, both parents must be included in the diagnostic study. Mother and father should be interviewed in the presence of their child, with each other in the absence of the child, and individually. These series of interviews should cover (1) the child's complete personal history, (2) the parents' marital history, (3) personal and family history of each parent, (4) the family culture, and (5) parental attitudes about causes and possible approaches to treatment or remedial measures.

Basic knowledge of the parents and family assists in understanding the dynamics of the child's illness. Family personalities and events are not always the cause of the symptoms, but they are always essential considerations in treatment and prognosis. The development of symptoms usually disrupts important interhuman relations, and disturbed relationships are often the cause of symptoms. Hence, many families at the time of examination have a self-feeding pathologic interaction system established. The natural dependency of the child makes his parents the most significant part of his environment. To attempt to diagnose or treat the child without the assistance of the parents or parent substitutes would be like trying to carry on treatment in a psychologic vacuum.

REFERENCES

1. Becker, W.C.: Consequences of different kinds of parental discipline, in *Review of Child Development Research,* Hoffman and Hoffman (Eds.). New York, Russell Sage Foundation, 1964, pp. 169–208.
2. Chess, S., Thomas, A., and Birch, H.: Behavior problems revisited. J. Am. Acad. Child Psychiatry, *6*:321, 1967.
3. Ehrenwald, J.: Neurosis in the family: a study of psychiatric epidemiology. Arch. Gen. Psychiatry, *3*:232, 1969.
4. ———: Family diagnosis and mechanisms of psychosocial defense. Family Proc., *2*:121, 1963.
5. ———: *Neurosis in the Family and Patterns of Psychosocial Defense.* New York, Hoeber, 1963.
6. Esalona, S.K. and Heider, G.M.: *Prediction and Outcome.* New York. Basic Books, Inc., 1959.
7. Gildea, M., Glidewell, J., and Kantor, M.: Maternal attitudes and general adjustment in school children, in *Parental Attitudes and Child Behavior,* Glidewell, J. (Ed.). Springfield, Ill., Charles C Thomas, 1961, p. 89.
8. Helper, M.M.: Parental evaluations of children and children's self-evaluations. J. Abnorm. Soc. Psychol., *56*:190, 1958.
9. Levitt, E.E.: A comparison of parental and self-evaluations of psychopathology in children. J. Clin. Psychol., *15*:402, 1959.
10. ———: Psychotherapy research and the expectation-reality discrepancy. Psychotherapy: Theory, Research and Practice, *3*:163, 1966.

11. Mark, J.C.: The attitudes of mothers of male schizophrenics toward child behavior. J. Abnorm. Soc. Psychol., *48*:185, 1953.

12. McAdoo, W.G.: The application of Goldberg's classification rules to parents in a child guidance clinic and in an adult psychiatric clinic. J. Community Psychol., *2*:174, 1974.

13. McAdoo, W.G. and Connolly, F.G.: MMPIs of parents in dysfunctional families. J. Consult. Clin. Psychol., *43*:270, 1975.

14. Robins, L.N.: Social correlates of psychiatric disorders: Can we tell causes from consequences? J. Health Soc. Behav., *10*:95, 1969.

15. ————: *Deviant Children Grown Up: A Sociological and Psychiatric Study of Sociopathic Personality.* Baltimore, Williams and Wilkins, 1966.

16. Rutter, M.: *Children of Sick Parents: An Environmental and Psychiatric Study.* London, Oxford University Press, 1966.

17. Sears, R.R., Macoby, E.E., and Levin, H.: *Patterns of Child Rearing.* Evanston, Ill., Row, Peterson and Co., 1957.

18. Shoben, E.J.: The assessment of parental attitudes in relation to child adjustment. Genet. Psychol. Monogr., *39*:101, 1949.

19. Simmons, J.E.: *Interviewing, in Ambulatory Pediatrics.* Green, M. and Haggerty, J. (Eds.). Philadelphia, W.B. Saunders and Co., 1968.

20. Tseng, W.W. and McDermott, J.F., Jr.: Triaxial family classification: A proposal. J. Am. Acad. Child Psychiatry, *18*:22, 1979.

21. Zuckerman, M. and Oltean, M.: Some relationships between maternal attitude factors and authoritarianism, personality needs, psychopathology, and self-acceptance. Child Dev., *30*:27, 1959.

22. Zuckerman, M., Barrett, B. and Bragiel, R.M.: The parental attitudes of parents of child guidance case. Child Dev., *31*:401, 1960.

9

THE CASE STUDY

A complete case study contains a past and present history of the child, a family history and an assessment of significant members of the child's current household, the psychologic test results, and the mental status report. A summation of these data should permit the clinical team or the individual clinician to make a diagnostic formulation and treatment plan for a particular child.

Some case material is presented here to illustrate the way our case study method leads to a diagnostic formulation. The formulation reflects the clinician's opinions regarding the type and severity of the emotional disorder, the most probable causes and contributing factors, and the course of treatment judged best for the patient. Admittedly, treatment is strongly influenced by the theoretical orientation of the clinician. Even so, theoretical constructs have to be adapted to the specific variety of disorder presented by the patient. The selection of which treatment for which child is dependent upon clinical judgment. Clinical acumen is continually influenced by the rapidly expanding body of knowledge regarding etiology and treatment methods.

In Chapter 7, the diagnostic formulation was defined as containing answers to the eight implicit questions about the child's adjustment level in his family. These questions guide the examiner in outlining the seriousness of the illness, the cause or causes, the treatment, and the prognosis.

Neither the history, the psychologic testing, nor the psychiatric examination alone can provide all of the answers to these questions. The history from the parents or guardians and the school give the parents' and teachers' views of the types and severity of impairments that they see in the child. The degree of illness and areas of relative health or impairment in the child's personality are more specifically identified by the psychologist's and psychiatrist's reports. Evidence for central nervous system impairment (question 3) is obtained from the history of birth, development, systems review, and past illnesses; from the physical and neurologic findings; and from the impressions of the psychologist and psychiatrist. The relevance of these findings to the presenting symptoms and personality configurations rests with clinical judgment. In a similar fashion, conclusions about the presence and relative importance of psychosocial factors are drawn from the history and from direct examinations, evaluated in the context of the clinician's current knowledge and hypotheses regarding psychopathogenesis.

The practice of establishing either a functional or an organic etiology has become passé. As diagnostic acumen has developed, clinicians are finding more and more cases in which both organic and functional factors appear to have been significant in the development of a particular disturbance. One or the other of these factors alone either would not have resulted in the development of disordered adjustment or would have resulted in a different symptom complex.

Similarly, as stated in Chapter 7, child psychiatrists have broadened their concept of functional etiology beyond the premise of the disturbed mother-child relationship. Experience has taught that the father-child relationships, mother-father interaction, or entire family interactions may be significant. Cultural and economic phenomena cannot be ignored, because of their influence on the configuration of family interaction patterns.

Multiple etiology is at least theoretically possible in every case and glaringly apparent in many. With this tenet the "either-or" concept of etiology is not very helpful clinically. The clinical concerns are summarized in questions 6 and 7 of the diagnostic formulation: How have the most probable causes converged to produce the symptom picture? Which of these contributing causes are still active and problematic to the situation? The answer to these questions leads to the final question of what can and must be done in the way of corrective procedures.

A diagnostic-treatment model can be illustrated by comparing child psychiatric treatment to some aspects of orthopedic surgery. The surgeon never "cures" a broken bone. He approximates the fragments and then places the injured part in a highly protective environment, the cast, to prevent further trauma or noxious agents from influencing the healing process. If the bone pathology is too severe or if healing fails to take place with conservative measures, he must then probe deeply into the seat of the pathology and attempt to make structural and other changes. At the risk of oversimplification, psychiatric treatment of children can be seen as an attempt insofar as possible to remove noxious and traumatic agents in order to permit healthy development to take place. Often psychotherapeutic effort to change ideas, feelings, and neurotic concepts is necessary for one or more members of the family. Whenever psychotherapy is used, concomitant manipulation of the immediate environment and a gradual resumption of normal functioning are always essential aspects of treatment. Injured bones and injured personalities never heal without scarring and some functional impairment. The ultimate goal of treatment is to achieve minimal disability. Successful treatment never provides insurance against future breaks under sufficient stress, but future problems can often be reduced if the degree of fragility of the organism is fully understood.

The case study outline that follows permits summarization of the evaluation data, yet is sufficiently inclusive and flexible to be applicable to a wide variety of conditions. The outline can be used to record the summary of relatively uncomplicated cases as well as to summarize the important information about children with multiple problems due to a diversity of causes.

Outline for Case Study

1. Identifying data

Name _____ Case No. _____

Address _____ Intake Date _____

Tel. No. _____ Race _____ Birth date _____ Age _____

School _____ Grade _____

Religion _____ Referred By _____

Natural Parents	Date	Current family	Name	Relation to patient	Age	Occupation or grade
Married	_____	Father	_____	_____	_____	_____
Separated	_____	Mother	_____	_____	_____	_____
Divorced	_____	Children (incl. patient)	_____	_____	_____	_____
Unknown	_____		_____	_____	_____	_____

Deceased family members

Relation to patient	Date of death	Cause of death	Age
_____	_____	_____	_____
_____	_____	_____	_____

Comments:

  2. Presenting problem:
  3. Course of symptoms and current adjustment of child (present illness):
  4. Family interaction and social picture:
  5. Preschool developmental history (includes prenatal history):
  6. Medical history (includes systems review plus past illnesses, injuries and operations):
  7. School history:
  8. Mother (personal history)
  9. Father (personal history):
 10. Child:
     A. Mental status examination
     B. Physical examination
     C. Special procedures
        (1) Laboratory
        (2) Psychologic test results
        (3) Consultation results
 11. Diagnostic formulation:
     A. Biopsychic-social dynamics and interaction of child and family
     B. DSM III diagnosis (use all five axes)
     C. Treatment plan
     D. "Contract" with family
 12. Follow-up visits (including parent conference):
 13. Treatment reviews:
     A. Current working diagnosis and progress in treatment
        1. The child
        2. The parents
     B. Recommendations for further treatment

On the following pages, three cases are presented in detail. The average clinician is confronted with a wide variety of psychiatric problems. The outline method of recording clinical data serves as a guide for the clinical case study and illustrates the process of case analysis and synthesis that is essential to treatment planning.

In our teaching programs all persons in training and new staff are required to use this case study outline for their patients' records. Although the outline has proved to be an excellent teaching device assuring completeness, it is time-consuming and not very cost-effective. Experienced staff use a shorter, condensed version of the outline.

In addition to the information required for the case summary outline, a school history is obtained directly from the child's school by using the following report form. A direct report from the school is particularly essential when the presenting complaint involves academic or social problem(s).

ACADEMIC AND BEHAVIORAL REPORT

Name _____ Grade _____ Date of birth _____

School _____ Address _____

Teacher's or counselor's name _____ Phone no. _____

Current grades (list subjects and most recent available grades):

1. _____   5. _____
2. _____   6. _____
3. _____   7. _____
4. _____   8. _____

Is child currently in danger of failing? Yes _____ No _____

Is child currently working close to capacity? Yes _____ No _____

Do current grades reflect improvement _____ decline _____ stability ____ in child's academic functioning during the past few months? Explain: _____

Check special instruction or placement: Recommended   Received

Special education class (Circle: gifted or retarded) _____

Repeat grade (list grade(s))   _____

Skip grade (list grade(s))   _____

Remedial reading   _____

Speech therapy   _____

Tutoring (list subject(s))   _____

If recommendations have been made, are such facilities available in present school? Yes _____ No _____ If not, where? _____

If child has special seating, indicate reason(s) by check: Eyesight _____ Hearing _____ Behavior _____ Other _____ . Explain: _____

Are you aware of or do you suspect any physical defects in child? Specify: ____

Comment on school adjustment:

Classroom behavior _____

Extra-classroom behavior (playground, lunchroom, etc.) _____

Attitude toward teachers _____

Peer relations _____

Personal habits and health _____

Attendance _____

Do these behaviors reflect improvement, decline or stability of this child's extra-academic functioning in the past few months? _____

Additional information (Please elaborate and use additional pages if needed):

1. Do other children in this family present problems?
2. Add any information about this child's home or family relationships that has a bearing on his school attitudes and behavior.
3. Are you aware of any previous evaluations that would provide further information?
4. Do you have any suggestions for helping this child?
5. Do you have any suggestions about how we might be of help to you?

_____

Signature of person completing report

_____   Date _____

Title

(Please provide results of formal standardized testing by completing the form on next page or by sending photocopies)

ACADEMIC AND BEHAVIORAL REPORT
Child's name _____

Intelligence test results

| | *When tested* | | |
Name of test	Date	Grade	Test results

Achievement test results

| | *When tested* | | | Grade | |
Name of test	Date	Grade	Subtest	Equivalent	Percentile

The preceding information can be mailed along with a signed release of information to the school. However, we obtain a nearly 100% return rate if we give the form with a self-addressed, stamped envelope to the parents and ask them to give it to the school teacher, counselor, social worker or other appropriate person.

REFUSAL TO ATTEND SCHOOL (SCHOOL PHOBIA)

Name: Jeffrey M.   Intake date: 2-20-66
Birth date: 8–29–59   Age: 6½ years
School: Consolidated Elementary
Religion: Protestant
Referred by: Family physician, Dr. N. B.

Family		Relation to patient	Age	Occupation or grade
Father	R.M.	Father	42	Machinist
Mother	E.M.	Mother	35	Homemaker
Children	F.M.	Sister	12	Sixth grade
	G.M.	Brother	10	Fourth grade
	J.M.	Patient	6½	First grade

Deceased Family Members

Paternal grandfather died in 1940 at age 65 after a stroke. Maternal grandmother died in the fall of 1965 at age 65 from a heart attack.

Presenting Problems

"He doesn't want to go to school." Since the death of his maternal grandmother 4 months ago, Jeff has not wanted to go to school. When he was sent to school, he just sat in his seat and cried for 2 hours or so until his parents were asked to come and take him home. If anyone tried to get him to work, he would become sassy. At home he is usually a very good boy, and the mother says, "He is a comfort to me because I need someone in the house with me." Only when an attempt is made to separate him from his mother does he become stubborn and angry.

Course of Symptoms and Current Adjustment of Child

Jeff started the first grade in September of 1965 at age 6. Both his mother and the school principal state that he was doing quite well and seemed to like school. In November Jeff contracted the measles. While he was home, the news came that Mrs. M.'s mother had died suddenly. Neither Jeff nor the other children seemed to be unduly disturbed by the news of their grandmother's death. The mother took it very hard and broke down and cried openly and frequently. By the time of the funeral, Jeff was almost well from the measles but was kept home from school another week. During this time the mother made daily trips to the maternal grandmother's (MGM's) grave and took Jeff with her. When Jeff was again sent back to school, he said he didn't want to go and upon arrival there just sat in his seat and cried. He told the teacher and his parents that he was afraid to go away from home because he thought his mother might not be there when he came back.

After a week or two of this behavior, he was removed from school on the advice of Dr. A. While he was at home with his mother, the daily trips to the M.G.M.'s grave were continued. The mother also consulted Dr. B., who told her to stop the daily trips to the grave and prescribed some nerve pills for her and a "white nerve medicine" for Jeff. Mrs. M. says that the nerve pills help her to some extent when she takes them, but that for quite a while Jeff would take his nerve medicine and spit it out in the bathroom. During this time she states that he was quite nervous and upset. He would jump up and down and shake all over in excitement but apparently enjoyed watching some TV programs (such as *Leave It to Beaver*). When she discovered he was not swallowing his nerve medicine, she forced him to swallow it in front of her and he became calmer. Mrs. M. was advised by her physician to try to wean Jeff from his dependence upon her by leaving him with friends for a few minutes at a time and by starting him into school a few minutes each day and increasing this time until he could stay there all day. She had little success with this program, however, and the boy has not gone back to school.

Jeff has continued to enjoy playing with his brother and sister and going to church and Sunday school with the family. Mrs. M. thinks that his behavior is improving slightly and that she herself is beginning to feel better in accepting her mother's death.

Background Information

Family Picture:

The family lives in a modern three-bedroom home built by the father in a rural area. The boys share one bedroom, each with his own bed, and the parents and sister have the other two. The two older children have continued in school and are seemingly unaffected by the present problem. The marriage has been generally harmonious, with mutual discussion of problems and plans. The mother is dissatisfied with the marriage in that she desires to have sexual relations more than once a week. She feels that her husband is inconsiderate in frequently forgetting to give her birthday, anniversary, and Christmas gifts. Their monthly payments for house, furniture, and car burden them so that she cannot afford to buy a set of false teeth. The MGM lived nearby, and Mrs. M. was often called upon to help her out when the grandmother was not feeling well. Mother also does cleaning work at their church and takes in ironing for pay in order to help supplement the family income and to keep herself busy.

Preschool Developmental History

Except for slight nausea and vomiting during the first 2 months, the pregnancy was normal until the last 2 months, when Mrs. M. states that she became so big that she could hardly walk because of pressure and pains down below. He was born 2 weeks late, weighing 8 pounds, 13½ ounces (2 pounds more than the other two children), after a 9-hour labor during which the pains were harder and quicker than those during the other pregnancies. The mother was given gas for the delivery and was told that he was born head first and everything was normal. Mother and child left the hospital the second day after birth, and she began to nurse him. She believes that her milk was not rich enough because he nursed all the time and she thought he was losing weight although he was not weighed. After 1 week of nursing he was changed to SMA formula, which he vomited, and then to Wilson formula, which he vomited, and finally when he was 10 days old she put him on straight homogenized milk, which agreed with him, and he thrived thereafter. Mother absolutely cannot recall when he sat up, walked, or began to talk, although she thinks these were at normal intervals. She states that he cried more than her other children, especially when she would leave the room or the house. Toilet training was started about 2 years of age, and it took only a few months to accomplish this. He has not been enuretic or incontinent since.

School History

See Course of Symptoms.

Medical History

He has had all immunizations. He had frequent respiratory infections until a year ago and measles in November of last year.

Mother

Mrs. M. is a plainly dressed woman of 35 who looks more like 50. She has a very sad expression on her face, no teeth, and readily talks of how sad she is and of how she believes that her friends and even her own sister do not care for her. She is the fifth in a family of eight children. She describes MGF as a good man who was strict and trained the children well. He was a farmer and also worked on the railroad section crew and did carpentry work on the side. He did not go to church with the family or to other activities with the children. She describes MGM as being a good woman, always giving to others (although not sacrificing her own needs). She took the children to church and was very happy when they joined.

The youngest child, Ellen, now 21, was her favorite. Ellen was born during the time when MGM was "in the change of life" and has always been sickly, having trouble with her stomach and nerves. All the mother's siblings except Ellen quit school because they didn't like it or wanted to get married. Only Ellen completed high school. Mrs. M. herself had to drop out of school at the age of 16 after completing the eighth grade in order to take care of MGM. MGM had been an ambitious, hardworking woman who liked to have large crowds of company, as many as 50 at a time. She was also sickly, with "rheumatism and arthritis"; when Mrs. M. was 16 these became so bad that she had to use crutches and a cane for about 6 months. Doctoring with home remedies such as lemon juice helped MGM become well enough to get rid of the crutches and cane. In spite of this, Jeff's mother still remained at home until she met her husband and married at the age of 19.

Mrs. M. has always been sensitive to criticism and even in the first grade would cry if scolded by the teacher. She has always regretted that she couldn't finish high school. She looks back on her childhood in the country and says that "life was better then than life is now." When her brother died in 1943, MGM had a "heart attack" and was sick in bed with trouble breathing for a week but did not go to the hospital.

The mother's description of meeting the father is as he gave it. She says that she was attracted to him because he was not smart or flirty like some boys. He didn't drink. He was good-looking and a steady worker. She says that they wanted four children but does not state a preference as to gender. She has enjoyed their sexual relations and achieves a climax each time. Though she wanted to have four children, the doctor told her that it would be too hard on her to have any more because Jeff had been so big that he had injured her too badly to allow her to have another child. After Jeff was born, they moved to their present house, which seemed too big to keep clean. She became afraid to whip and discipline the children because she thought she might hurt them. During this time she also cried a lot and was given some nerve pills, which she took for a month or two. She feels very gloomy and blue for a couple of days before each period. About 4 years ago she went through several months during which she had cramping low abdominal pains prior to each menstrual period, and exploratory surgery was performed. Her appendix was removed, and she was told that she had pinworms in it. A cyst was also removed from one ovary, though the doctor said there was no danger from this. She has not had abdominal pain since.

The mother says that she has again begun to cry more during the past year. She has also felt that their friends and even her sister do not really care for her and has felt more acutely her husband's neglect of anniversaries and birthdays. She was quite grieved by the death of her mother and says it was a comfort to have Jeff home with her. On the other hand, she feels that if he had not been home with the measles the first week after her mother's death she would have been able to "work out my problems better myself."

About June or July of 1965 (10 months ago) she had a severe headache from "sinus trouble." She felt that life was not worth living, that she would just like to go to bed and get away from it all and cry all day. She wanted to die but has not thought of suicide since then. She sleeps well and has no trouble with going to sleep at night or waking up in the middle of the night. About 2 years ago she had one bad dream, which she blames on her nerves. She felt that all the walls of the room were closing in on her and she couldn't escape. She also worries about family finances. She feels that she takes everybody's worries on herself.

Mrs. M.'s insight into her own and Jeff's problems is slight, though by the second interview she stated that perhaps the problem might be her "nerves" and not just Jeff's being stubborn and not wanting to go to school. It is the examiner's impression that the mother is a rather dependent person, always closely tied to MGM, striving to please her and other authority figures, having sacrificed her education for her mother and suffering rivalry with the favored younger sister. She seems to be moderately depressed at this time and has shown symptoms of depression ever since Jeff's birth.

Father

Mr. M., age 42, is the youngest in a family of six, including two half siblings by a former marriage of his mother. He is a plain man dressed in working clothes who states that he does not like to come to Metropolis because he always gets lost in the big city. (On visits to the clinic the family is brought by a sister of Mrs. M. who lives in the suburbs and drives them across the city.) Paternal grandfather (PGF) is described as a "typical old farmer" who barely made enough to get by on a 20-acre farm in spite of being a very hard worker. He was described as very kindhearted. He was relatively easygoing in comparison to the paternal grandmother (PGM) but was able to keep law and order among the children by use of a razor strap or belt. PGM is described as the one who had the drive in the family. PGM took all the children to church every week, though PGF seldom went. The father cannot describe any particular closeness to either one of his parents.

Mr. M. seems to have had a relatively uneventful boyhood, riding horses, playing ball, going hunting, going on hay rides with the young people from the church, and attending movies for entertainment. Of course, he had to work hard on the farm as well. He enjoyed school and made fairly good grades. He took all the courses in Latin offered at his school and wanted to go on to further courses but could not because they did not teach them. During his junior year in high school his father died of kidney trouble, and the next spring he had to quit school and get a job "in order to have enough to eat." His two full sisters who are just a few years older than he were able to complete high school. He went to work as a farm hand and had various jobs until called into the army near the end of the World War II. He completed training just in time to spend 18 months in the Army of Occupation as an MP. He went around with some of the German girls but "did not do the things that many of the other soldiers were doing with them." Upon his return from the army, he asked a friend for a job as a carpenter. He worked for this man for several years until asked to go to the city to build houses. He thought this was too far away and didn't like big cities, so he quit and got another job in his home area. At the time of his marriage in 1951 he was working for a coal yard but lost his job the week after he was married. After a few weeks of hunting, he went back to working for the original carpenter and has worked for him for the past 15 years in his home town.

Mr. M. says he met his wife in a movie theater one evening. When asked what attracted him to marry her he said, "That is a very hard question; I don't know." He says that now he appreciates her because she is a good cook and takes good care of the children. He courted his wife by taking her to the movies, going to visit the neighbors, driving in the countryside, and going to ball games. He can remember proposing to her while driving one Sunday but cannot remember anything that he said or she said. They had no plans for the number or sex of children they wanted prior to marriage. He says their sexual adjustment was satisfactory and that now intercourse once a week is enough for him although during the earlier years of their marriage he was "more of a man." He was willing to have "as many children as the good Lord would give" but also feels that it is about time to stop now.

It is the impression of the interviewer that Mr. M. is a plain, simple man. His ego strength seems to be adequate to meet the needs of his situation, limited as it is, though he admits that he cannot stand the stresses of the larger world around him and goes to pieces when he comes into the city and gets lost in traffic. His affect was appropriate. He seemed somewhat uncomfortable with the examiner, though he was cooperative and able to respond. In the joint interview of the family he seemed to offer little support to his wife in her explanation of her emotional problems. He does take an active part in the affairs of the home, playing ball and other games with the children and disciplining them when he is there. He takes the family to church nearly every Sunday and is happy that the children are showing interest in it. His insight into Jeff's and the family's problems is quite limited, though he realizes that the main problem of not wanting to go to school is related to his wife and her grief over her mother's death. One recent sign of awareness of his wife's need for support is the fact he gave her a box of candy at Valentine's Day this year, which was a complete surprise to her and made her very happy.

Mental Status Examination

Jeff was neatly dressed in a blue suit, in contrast to the plain clothing of his parents. He appeared sad and stood clinging to his mother in the waiting room. When it was suggested that he come along to play, he became sullen with downcast eyes and said, "I won't go." His mother was invited to the examining room with us. Jeff immediately showed interest in the toys but then refused to play and sat with arms folded on a chair. When the mother was invited to leave the room, he suggested the alternative of playing with the toys in the hall, where his mother was taking her MMPI test. On the second visit he readily and happily accepted leaving his mother to go and play. While in the room, he said several times, "That other room didn't have as many toys in it as this one" and "The reason children don't like to play so well the first time is because they don't know how much fun it is at the clinic."

Jeff's orientation and perception are good. Neuromuscular integration is normal. Thought processes are orderly and he verbalizes well. Intelligence seems to be average. His fantasy play and other comments show a preoccupation with people being hurt or killed, especially the mother. He spontaneously began drawing a brown figure in the shape of a house, which he said was a mountain with rocks falling off it, crushing the cars below and hurting the people. He also commented that the dollhouse looked as if a tornado had hit it. He said it was dangerous to live on the edge of the table as the people in the dollhouse did because they might be hit by a tornado. He was frequently distracted by the sound of sirens, saying that the ambulance was going to pick up sick people who had been hurt in an accident, or there were fire trucks, or that they might be going to pick up sick people or going to an accident. He said they saw a wreck on the way home in which someone was killed, and his mother had seen a car rolled over on the way today. While playing with the truck, moving the furniture out of the dollhouse, he put a baby in the house, saying that it might get hit by the truck. He went on to say that the mother might also be hit by the truck and die. Then the family would have no mother.

He fired the gun and said he wished he could have one but that his mother wouldn't let him have any because she was afraid of guns. He drew a picture of a boat, and though he could not see the people on it he made up a story about a family there. He said the people were happy on the boat, but some might be sad because they couldn't get up on top and pilot the boat for fear of being thrown off and drowned. This would make the family sad, and they would "kick other people" and then cry. He expressed the thought that if the baby were kicked he might die or if the husband were kicked he might kick back at the mother. He said that the boy might help his mother if she were sad by staying home or by buying presents for her instead of going outside and playing.

He said his favorite television show was *Casper the Ghost*. He said that Casper had no friends and was always trying to make friends but whenever they found out he was a ghost they would be scared away. He also related a TV story about a rocket ship that crashed and resulted in injury for the occupants. His three wishes were for material things: to have a gun like the one in the playroom, to have a car of his own, and to have another car, a pick-up truck. He asked me to copy a picture of a bear from a book, and as I was doing it he said, "Make it sad," although the bear in the book had a smile. When asked why the bear was sad, he said, "Mommy won't let him have a gun." When drawing a person he drew a vague figure and first said it was a mom and later said it was a little girl who was in a bear costume for Halloween.

Jeff appears to be struggling with the fear that he will not grow up to be a man. His desire to break away from the mother's dominance is shown by his interest in masculine playthings and in his ability to leave her happily at the second visit. His fear of separation would appear to be largely a reaction formation against hostility aroused by conflict with the mother. However, his grandmother's death and the mother's current depression give his fear of her injury or death some reality basis. His play indicates a constant concern about catastrophe. He has some awareness of mother's depression and feels he should try to help her.

Diagnostic Conference

Formulation

Jeff's main symptom is separation anxiety. The mother appears to have been a rather self-effacing woman all her life, dependent for approval on the maternal grandmother, in particular, but less favored than her sickly younger sister. She has shown symptoms of depression at least since Jeff's birth, compounded recently by the death of MGM. She would appear to regard Jeff ambivalently as the child who was hard to bear and ended her childbearing capability yet as the person from whom she must receive support and approval now that MGM is gone. The mother holds him close and is afraid to let him go. The father is a rather dependent person, able to function only in his unchanging, simple home community; and incapable of giving his wife the amount of support and approval she needs. Jeff appears to be ready to break away from his mother's dominance. The mother seems to desire help with her feelings of inadequacy and dependency and should be able to benefit from therapy.

The father shows little interest in help for himself but may possibly be encouraged to support the mother a little more than he has in the past.

DSM III Diagnosis

This case was evaluated nearly 16 years before the publication of *DSM III*. From the preceding case material we offer:

Axis I: 309.21—Separation anxiety disorder
Axis II: V71.09—No diagnosis
Axis III: No physical disorder
Axis IV: 4: Moderate; absence from school for measles, death of maternal grandmother; chronic maternal depression
Axis V: Adaptive functioning past year: 2, very good; school, peer and family adjustment was satisfactory prior to the onset on the anxiety

Conference Recommendations

1. Jeff is very ready for active play sessions that would involve handling his feelings concerning aggression and dependency. He particularly needs to express and better understand his relationship with his mother, whom he sees as not allowing him to grow up and "use guns."
2. Mrs. M. should be seen in therapy by a therapist who might offer her support, initially recognize the frustration of her dependency needs, and gradually help her to turn to her husband and perhaps those outside her home for such satisfaction. It is difficult to determine at this point how much insight this woman may gain into her depression. Antidepressant medication for mother was considered but deferred.
3. The father should be seen only occasionally and then probably with his wife and her therapist in an effort to help him be more giving and supportive of the wife.
4. Jeff should return to school immediately. The principal should be contacted and urged to allow the child to attend school even though he may not be able to pass the first grade. He should stay the entire school day and, if he becomes upset, be allowed to go to the principal's office until he regains control and once again can return to the classroom. The child should come to the disposition conference and be reassured that he can go to school and that his mother will be there when he gets home.

(Signed) Conference Chairman

Contract with Family

Mr. and Mrs. M. were approximately 1 hour late because of Mr. M's fear of driving in the city. The mother accepted very easily the idea that she was depressed and that it was her need to have the child home that was precipitating and intensifying the boy's school phobia. She accepted individual treatment for herself. Jeff has returned to school. Again, it seems quite apparent that the mother's concerns are most important in this area. She was very worried about how much he will cry at school. The father was supported in his desire to have the child help him do carpentry work around the house, such as building a dog house for a new stray dog Jeff had found. Treatment hour at 1:00 p.m. or morning would be best for the family.

Treatment Conference (Three Months after the Diagnosis Conference)

Current Working Diagnosis and Progress in Treatment:

Child

Jeff has been seen for 12 hours during the past 3 months. Initially he was tense and shaky. He tried to get me involved in games such as pool with him but was so tense that he couldn't play. For instance, at pool he couldn't hold the cue steady enough to shoot. I discouraged him from the game and gave him more physical distance. The overt anxiety cleared after several sessions. He then became demanding, seeking gifts and gratifications. He wanted to take various toys home. He always wanted to go to another office to find a toy different from what was present in my office. When restricted to my office and the toys therein, he accepted the restriction and now is less demanding. He plays with the burp guns and dart guns, shooting at the targets on the door. He plays with the building blocks, trucks, softball, and bat. He usually plays by himself and verbalizes happenings at home and things that he has done. At some time during the therapy hours he gets me involved in his games.

Each time there has been a siren outside, Jeff has commented "There goes another ambulance." When I asked him more about this he changed the subject quickly, until recently he said that he saw an ambulance on the road with someone inside it. He then said it made him think of his grandmother, who died in November. He said that the doctor hadn't arrived there in time to save his grandmother. Each time he heard the ambulance he thought of that and hoped the doctor would get there to save whoever was hurt. He didn't know why the doctor hadn't been there to save his grandmother, but the doctor was a slowpoke. He denied anger about the doctor. Several therapy hours later, when Jeff commented on a siren he heard, I asked him whether he were feeling bad when he heard the sirens. He replied, "I don't get that feeling anymore. I just say phooey on grandma. She's dead. What's the use of thinking about her? She can't come back to life. I don't even dream about her anymore. Besides, who would want to go through one of those spells again? You know, that spell about grandma."

Jeff has always avoided talking about his mother and any worries he may have about her or the rest of the family. He discussed having to take the first grade over and seems to have accepted it. He said he didn't fail and he didn't pass. They just wanted him to take it over because he missed so much school. He says he doesn't care, because he will learn more anyway.

The report from school indicates regular attendance and improvement in his relations with both peers and adults. His attention span and attitude toward his studies are improving. However, he will be retained in the first grade because he has missed too much to make up the work.

In summary, I think Jeff has made some progress, at least in therapy hours. He is less overtly anxious and more independent and has ventilated a lot of feelings. Although he uses denial extensively about his mother, he verbalizes some insight regarding grandmother's death.

Mother

She is without reservation in coming for help for herself and recognizes that there is a connection between her problems and Jeff's problems. Initially she expressed much emotion in the hours, talking about her anger at the demands people make upon her, especially a very disturbed, neglected neighbor child. After this was somewhat resolved, there was a plateau for a few weeks in April and May. When we began talking about her treatment of Jeff as a special child, this opened the subject of her relationship to MGM and the dam broke. For a number of weeks we have discussed her feelings of loss since MGM's death. She has worked through a great many feelings and is very busily involved in church and family activities. She is a very simple rural woman who seems to have low average intelligence, is not superstitious, but tends to use somewhat illogical cause-and-effect reasoning. She has agreed that she should come for treatment even if Jeff discontinues his treatment. She is aware of a great deal of improvement in both the boy and herself.

Conference Recommendations

Jeff is symptom-free at this time. The boy has quite satisfactorily worked through his feelings about his grandmother's death. Although he is unable to talk in therapy about his mother, he no longer clings to her or she to him. It may be necessary to explore more fully his relations with his parents. However, in view of his current freedom from anxiety and the fact his therapist is leaving the clinic, we will discontinue therapy for the time being.

Mrs. M. is currently discussing her relationship with her mother and is progressing satisfactorily. She should continue at least a few more sessions until she has better insight into her feelings about her mother.

(Signed) Conference Chairman

Final Treatment Conference (Approximately 6 months after the beginning of therapy)

Since the last treatment review, Mrs. M. has been seen for an additional 11 sessions at weekly intervals and a final session after a lapse of 6 weeks. She discussed her earlier relationships with her mother and her current feelings about her siblings. She has become quite direct—at times, almost impulsive—in verbalizing her anger to the therapist, to her husband, and to her siblings.

She has become able to hold her own in family arguments without excessive guilt, and her depression has abated. Her excessive somatization has lessened and she now follows her doctor's advice. Recent part-time employment out of the home has contributed much to her sense of well-being.

Both parents and school report Jeff to be doing well. Case closed. No further treatment needed.

(Signed) Conference Chairman

ASSAULTIVE BEHAVIOR IN A 7-YEAR-OLD

Name: Granville A.   Intake date: 5/17/67
Birth date: 12/29/59   Age: 7½ years
School: Lyman Elementary
Religion: Protestant
Referred by: Family physician, Dr. A. W.

Family	Relation to patient		Age	Occupation or grade
Father	Unknown			
Mother	Mary A.	Mother	29	Unemployed
Children	Granville	Patient	7½	First grade
	Ellen	Half-sister	3	
	Sybille	Half-sister	2	

Others Living in the Home

Maternal grandmother, age 52
Stepmaternal grandfather, age 59

Presenting Problem

Behavior problems at home and school. Until 4 months ago was in parochial school, where he choked, pinched, and jumped on other children. Obeys the teacher but not for long.

Course of Symptoms and Current Adjustment of Child

The patient is a 7½-year-old Black male. His mother dates the onset of present difficulty to about 4 months ago. Actually it was at this time that the mother realized the magnitude of the child's problem.

In March of this year, the mother received a call from the parochial school and was informed of his expulsion. The person who called indicated to the mother that the patient had been involved in numerous fights and had been observed kicking, fighting, and choking other students. It was felt by the school that the patient should be transferred to another facility.

The mother states that this all came as quite a shock to her. Although she knew her son was having some difficulty academically in school, she had no idea of the aggressive behavior of which she was told. The child was then transferred to the Lyman Public School, where he was assigned a male teacher. School reports indicate that he related rather well to this individual. His grades, however, were such that he is being retained in the first grade.

Granville is the oldest of three children, having two half-sisters, ages 3 and 2. His mother has never been married. She states that Granville has always been "a mischievous child," but she has never considered him to be bad. However, Granville did attempt to punch the baby off his mother's lap and take the baby's bottle. He would say on occasion, "Mama, you don't need that baby; I'm your baby." The patient in recent years seemed to have adapted quite well to his half-sisters and plays with them.

The patient's mother and half-sisters came to this area approximately 2 years ago at the insistence of MGM. The patient was originally enrolled at the parochial kindergarten because "they taught religion" and "they had a school bus so he wouldn't have to walk." Apparently he was believed to be ready for first grade, having had no difficulty in kindergarten.

The mother describes the patient as having a hot temper. He gets angry quite easily whenever things don't go his way. Frequently, he cries when frustrated. He can offer no reasons to her about his difficulties with other children. Also the mother indicates that the patient, who was toilet trained by 2 years of age, has been enuretic at a frequency of every other night for the past 6 or 7 months.

Background Information

Family Picture

The family is currently composed of Granville, his mother Mary, and two half-sisters, all of whom reside with the maternal grandmother and the maternal step-grandfather. The patient's maternal uncle also lives with his family in the same town. There are several male cousins to whom Granville is rather close. Step-grandfather is a laborer. Mother receives welfare assistance for her children.

Preschool Developmental History

Delivery was at home and was apparently uncomplicated. The patient had the usual childhood diseases but has had no serious illnesses requiring hospitalization. He sat at 3 to 4 months of age and walked at 11 months. He was toilet trained by 2 years of age. He has been enuretic for the past 6 months. He also talks a great deal in his sleep and has for some time.

School History

See Course of Symptoms.

School Report

"Much better behavior since transfer to public school and a male teacher. Although attendance good, he was absent the days achievement tests were given. However, in spite of improved conduct he has not grasped the basic academic skills and will be retained in the first grade. Mother seems distant and uninterested."

Medical History

There are no significant medical illnesses in the patient's past history.

Mother

Mary A. is a 29-year-old Black female. She has an obvious physical deformity, a severe right scoliosis with elevation of the right scapula, making her quite short and giving her a humpbacked appearance.

Miss A. was the third of five children. She was born June 22, 1937. She has brothers 4 and 2 years older, and 2 and 4 years younger. The family originally lived in the South, and the patient's mother started school there. When she was 6 or 7 years of age, the maternal grandfather ran off with another woman. Maternal grandmother moved with her family to another state after that. Miss A., who had completed 2 years of grade school, was put back and had to start all over again. Apparently she had no difficulty in school until approximately 11 years of age. At that time she fell from a tree and "my spine started growing crooked." At about 13 years of age doctors put her into a brace. After that (the mother cannot remember exactly when) she was taken to Memphis, Tennessee, where she underwent surgery, following which she wore a body cast. However, when the cast was removed, the scoliotic condition was unchanged and even worsened. During this period Miss A. became disgusted with everything and wanted to quit school. However, at her mother's insistence, she continued high school and graduated at age 19.

Miss A. enrolled in a state university but remained for only 1 year. She states that she couldn't make it academically. She then enrolled in a trade school. While still enrolled in school, she became pregnant with the patient. She states that the father promised to marry her but he didn't. She became quite disgusted and eventually quit school. The patient was born in December 1959. Miss A. states that prior to the pregnancy she knew very little of sex, having learned everything she knew from other girls. Her mother used to talk to her prior to that only in terms of staying away from men. The mother tried various types of pills in order to get her menstrual period started but made no active attempt to abort herself when pregnant with Granville. She states that she definitely did not want the pregnancy but accepted it. She went to live with her oldest paternal uncle and his wife and continued living there after the birth of the patient. She shared babysitting chores with the uncle's wife and was able at times to get out of the house. When Granville was 5 years of age, his mother became pregnant by another man. She states that she loved this man and thought that he would marry her. She has had three children but no marriage. Approximately 2½ years ago, the mother was asked by the maternal grandmother to come live here. MGM had remarried when the mother was approximately 15 years of age. MGM has given her "hell" for having three illegitimate children and for failing her (MGM). Miss A. states that this used to upset her and make her quite angry but that now she simply ignores MGM.

MGM is described as a "good lady. She raised all five of us without a daddy." However, MGM continues to dominate the home. Maternal step-grandfather is described as a good, quiet man "who has tried to help me as much as he can."

Mother started training in a vocational rehabilitation program about 2 weeks ago. She states that at first she didn't think she would be able to make it and this upset her a great deal. However, now she feels she can make it.

She related in a rather distant manner, showing little evidence of anxiety or concern. There is a great deal of psychomotor retardation, but she denies being depressed. On direct questioning she states she feels the fact that Granville is Black may have had something to do with the trouble he had in school. She indicates that other children in that school system who are Black have complained of being intimidated by White youths.

Father

All information about the father was obtained from the mother. She states that Granville's father now lives in the South. She feels that Granville knows who his father is because, while they lived near him, the father sometimes stopped Granville on the street and gave him money. She has never talked to the patient about his father, although he has asked frequently. The mother's only description of the father is that he was a drinking man who apparently had some difficulty learning in school.

Mental Status Examination

Granville was examined on three occasions. He was initially seen with his mother in a joint interview. He was also observed by me on several occasions while he was in the lobby in the child guidance clinic, as well as being seen for two individual playroom sessions at weekly intervals.

On each occasion, Granville was quite neat in appearance. He rapidly scanned his surroundings in most instances. He appeared to be a bright youngster with a great deal of curiosity. Especially noteworthy was the ease with which he was able to leave his mother. In fact, he often was completely oblivious to her presence. At the time of the initial interview, he shook hands with the examiner. He sat in a chair only a short time before he was up inspecting my office. He immediately picked up a dart gun and loaded it. He then called, "Mother!" When she turned around, he pointed the gun at her but did not shoot.

Granville was well oriented for the most part. However, at the initial interview, he said he was told he was going to an eye doctor. When informed of who I was, he simply nodded but offered no comment. Granville said that he was going to be retained in the first grade because he was bad, yet he could offer no source of this information. Throughout each interview, he continually shot darts either at the target on the door or at dominoes that he had lined up on the bookshelf. He often answered questions with his back to the examiner.

He is well coordinated. His speech is usually coherent, although at times it is difficult to hear. He described a recurrent nightmare in which a black humpbacked man was going to kill him. His drawings of a man and woman were rather bizarre, with little attention paid to body form and appendages. His drawing of a woman, in fact, was quite poor. He wishes that (1) he could have a horse so that he could ride around the country, (2) he could have a cowboy suit and be a western boy so that he could shoot with a real gun, and (3) he could have a real gun so that he could show it to people and shoot it up in the sky. "I'm a good shot. Got to be good shot by chunkin' rocks." When questioned about his mother, he would only say, "Ain't got nothing to say about her. She comes out and plays with me sometimes." He immediately began talking about guns again after this interchange. He volunteered that he sleeps in the lower bunk with his mother because he fears falling out of the top bunk. He would not talk about his sisters. When he was finished playing, he left toys and darts on the floor. However, when reminded of this, he immediately picked them up. It is my feeling that he will respond when limits are set, but this has probably not been done consistently in the past.

Granville feels that he must have been bad because he is being retained in the first grade. Yet in his fantasy he would like to be one of the good guys. He talks about being a sheriff or a policeman and chasing bad boys.

In summary, this 7½-year-old Black male is quite neat in appearance. He seems preoccupied with thoughts of aggressiveness and constantly acts these out. He also seems to be preoccupied with the idea of his own badness. He appears to be of average intelligence. There appears to be a great deal of difficulty with self-identity. Also there are indications of a poor concept of women as exemplified by his mother, with whom he is quite angry.

Psychologic Testing

Tests Administered

Draw-A-Person Test
Wechsler Intelligence Scale for Children
Thematic Apperception Test
Structured Doll Play Technique

Granville is a nice-looking 7½-year-old Black boy, who was tested at the request of Dr. L. Consultation was requested primarily concerning the following questions: (1) intellectual level, (2) ability to handle aggressive impulses, (3) awareness of own difficulties, and (4) ability to work in therapy with a male therapist. Granville was cooperative although somewhat slow during the testing session, and he seemed to relate rather well to this examiner.

The predominant impression from the test material is that Granville is involved in a rather difficult and confusing relationship with his mother. He feels that to please her, he must be strong and responsible or his mother will reject and/or leave him. He also feels pressured from his mother to meet some of her needs. Granville finds it quite difficult to satisfy his mother, and he feels inadequate to meet her expectations. His feelings of inadequacy are also contributed to by his perception of adult males as ineffectual and distant; he has apparently been unable to identify with an adequate male figure.

Although he tries to satisfy his mother by being a little man, at times his dependency needs become quite strong, and he feels that his mother does not try to meet them. Although feeling attached to her (perhaps neurotically so), he is quite angry at the emotional distance perceived between himself and her. As long as he is the little man, he and his mother have an adequate relationship, but when he demands dependency-need gratification, he also fears rejection. Hence, he is reluctant to express his anger about his ungratified dependency needs directly toward his mother and vents his hostility on others. For example, he is quite hostile toward other children. In addition, his feelings of inadequacy have been exacerbated by his experiences in school, where he feels he is rejected and scorned. The only controls over the expression of his hostility that were prominent in test data are denial and suppression, and these become inadequate rather readily; hence, aggressive outbursts are probably easily elicited from him.

With the many burdens and frustrations that Granville perceives in real life, he finds some gratification in active fantasy. Although some slightly autistic fantasy was manifested in his Rorschach responses, this was not sufficiently bizarre to suggest psychosis. He does appear to be at least moderately emotionally disturbed, with his difficulties' being primarily of a neurotic and characterologic nature. The amount, availability, and poor control of his hostility indicate that psychotherapy is necessary for him at this time. He appears to be a bright, sensitive boy, in spite of his history of poor school performance. Although he achieved an IQ score of only 91 on the Wechsler Intelligence Scale for Children, his talent for reasoning and sizing up situations seems indicative of above-average intellectual capacity. In addition, Granville does appear to feel discomfort about himself and his situation. Thus he appears to have talents and motivation that would be positive assets in psychotherapy.

Diagnostic Formulation

This 7½-year-old Black male was referred to this clinic for evaluation because of outbursts of aggressive behavior directed toward peers and because of difficulty in school. He is the oldest of three children of his unwed mother. The patient's mother has a severe physical deformity and some disability. Granville was an unwanted child, but after his birth his mother devoted her entire attention to him. However, the mother has remained chronically unhappy, and it appears that she is constantly unable to satisfy the boy's needs. The mother became pregnant again 5 years after his birth. His reaction to this was one of extreme hostility, which he has been unable to control adequately. His behavior at school represents an expression of hostility. Also, because of cultural variables, this child was not prepared for entrance into the school situation. The lack of a father figure is confusing to him and has given him no one with whom to identify. The mother clinically appears detached, distant, and somewhat suspicious of the motives of others. Granville's problems at this time represent a behavior disorder that assumes a characterologic pattern. However, fixed patterns do not seem well established yet. The mother's personal and social problems and the current living situation are continuous stimulants of his aggressive behavior and deprive him of controls and identification models.

Diagnosis

DSM II—308.4—Unsocialized aggressive reaction of childhood.

Treatment Recommendations

1. Granville is an attractive Black boy with many social and cultural strikes against him. He needs an adequate masculine figure with whom to identify. He seems to be seeking ways to express himself more appropriately and be accepted. He will be seen weekly by a male therapist. In addition, we will explore the resources in his community for group recreative experiences outside the home. (Now, some 18 years later, Ritalin or one of the major tranquilizers might be used in addition to his psychotherapy.)
2. Miss A. should have an evaluation of her physical deformity. In view of the many advances in orthopedic surgery in the past 20 years, a current evaluation is needed. Miss A. will also be seen weekly at this clinic. She will no doubt resist exploration of her feelings and personal relationships. Help will be offered with her medical and vocational problems and in matters of the home management of Granville. If a trusting relationship can be established, it may be possible to explore her problems with her mother and with men. However, at this time she truly needs aggressive casework assistance with her reality problems.

Disposition Conference

Miss A. was seen and the staff recommendations were reviewed with her. She readily accepted the idea of weekly therapy sessions for Granville. She was a bit more reluctant about sessions for herself but agreed to come. She accepted an appointment for evaluation by the orthopedic department. First therapy session scheduled for 2:00 p.m. on August 20.

Summary of Therapy

In therapy, Granville rather quickly formed a very positive attachment to his therapist. In play-acting he reviewed many of his conflicts about his mother and himself. School behavior improved both socially and academically. However, at home he continued to be caught in the conflicts of the mother and grandmother.

It required intensive casework to help Miss A. overcome her extreme pessimism and accept rather extensive and prolonged orthopedic treatment. Upon learning that Miss A. would require extended bed care, a conference was arranged with her, the grandmother, the local public health nurse and the welfare department to plan for her convalescence and the continued care of the children. Arrangements were made for Granville to be placed in a group home where he could continue receiving psychotherapy. The grandmother agreed to continue to provide a home for the mother and sisters with assistance from the public health nursing service.

Granville had some difficulty adjusting initially in the group home, but he rather quickly made good progress in his behavior and his relations with others. Remedial education was not available, but he made B's and C's in school even though the standardized achievement tests showed him somewhat below his age level.

He was discharged from the home to his mother after a residence of 3 years, 2 months. After the extensive orthopedic treatment his mother's health improved and she was employed part-time. Granville had to have some remedial help during high school, but there were no disciplinary problems at home or school, and no delinquency was reported. The record is not clear regarding graduation from high school. He left home shortly after his eighteenth birthday, which his mother considered appropriate. A few months later a report was received from another state that he was shot to death in a stolen car during a high-speed chase by the sheriff. To the best of our knowledge this was the first time Granville had ever violated the law. We have only newspaper reports and a verbal account from his mother. Unknown are the details of the auto theft and why violent means were needed to stop him. We cannot say to what extent sociologic factors or his own psychopathology was responsible for his untimely death.

SCHOOL FAILURE OF AN 8-YEAR-OLD

Name: __Jimmy D.__   Intake date: 10/5/78
Birth date: __8/2/70__   Age __8 years__
School: __Escalante Elementary__
Religion: __Protestant__
Referred by: __Dr. L, the mother's psychiatrist__

	Family	Relation	Age	Occupation
Father	Harold D.	Father	28	Laborer
Mother	Sylvia D.	Mother	28	Secretary
Children	Jimmy D.	Patient	8	Second
	No siblings			grade

Presenting Problem

Problem with school, i.e., failing courses.

Course of Symptoms and Current Adjustment of Child

The parents state that Jimmy has had to repeat the first grade in school, did poorly during his repeat year, and is now doing very poorly in the second grade. Mrs. D. discussed her concern about Jimmy's school problem with her psychiatrist, who referred the family to this clinic.

Jimmy began first grade at age 6 and did poorly from the beginning. He brought home papers with poor grades but was not involved in any disciplinary problems or absenteeism. The mother states that she was not overly concerned at the time because she felt that perhaps Jimmy was still a little bit too young to accept the full responsibilities for achieving in school. He failed virtually every course and after repeating the first grade was promoted to the second grade because of "social pressure" and because the teacher "wanted to get rid of him." With further questioning, the parents also reported that Jimmy has problems relating to other children. He is unable to form close or lasting friendships because he imposes overly strong demands on his friends in play activity, and when they do not abide by his demands he becomes violently angry with them.

Both the mother and father feel that a poor family environment and two episodes of acute psychotic reactions in the mother have contributed most significantly to Jimmy's problems. The father is, however, considerably more outspoken about this. Both parents express guilt feelings and now want to compensate him for all the "lack of love" that he experienced during the more turbulent periods of their relationship. They do this primarily by not imposing disciplinary limits on the child. When he does transgress the few behavioral limits they have for him, they do not punish him. The father states that during the first episode of acute psychosis that the mother suffered, she attempted to handle the school problem by "beating Jimmy." Father states that she would beat him so viciously with a belt that he would bleed from the wounds on his back. This did not continue very long, as the father would not allow it. Jimmy developed an overt fear of his mother that persists to the present. The father states that the child often begged not to be left alone with the mother, as he was afraid of what she would do to him. The more recent attempts by the parents to handle this school problem have been primarily by helping with schoolwork. This, however, has not proved successful.

The parents still argue about discipline. The father feels that Jimmy should have more rigid behavioral limitations than he does but that he should not be punished physically for misbehavior. The mother, on the other hand, feels that Jimmy should not be limited by strict behavioral controls, and when he does misbehave she spanks him very severely with a belt. The parents observed Jimmy playing with his genitals about 1 year ago. This behavior continued, and the father admonished him not to do it. The mother's approach to this was one of "educating him," and she states that she explained to Jimmy the physiology of reproduction. Jimmy has been sleeping with his mother during the past year while father has been working the night shift. According to the father, Jimmy says that his mother makes him sleep with her.

Background Information

Family Picture

The father is currently employed as a laborer of somewhat above the minimum wage. The mother is employed as a typist at a small store at minimum wage. The family lives in a five-room rented home. The family does not share in any activity together. There appears to be no positive interaction between the mother and father or between the mother and Jimmy. The significant interaction that does occur in this family appears to be limited to the relationship between Jimmy and his father.

Preschool Developmental History

Mrs. D. became pregnant about 1 year after the marriage, and both parents state that although the pregnancy was not planned they were desirous of having a child in the near future and therefore the fact of the pregnancy was well accepted. The pregnancy and delivery were uneventful. Jimmy's birth weight was 8 pounds, 6 ounces, and the immediate postnatal course was uneventful. There were no birth defects or difficulties with eating or development. Jimmy sat up at about 6 months, talked at 9 months, walked at 16 months, and was toilet trained at about 2 years.

School Report

"Jimmy daydreams and plays instead of doing his work. Repeated first grade. Now in second grade placement, but achievement is near failure. California Mental Maturity Test last year rated IQ level as average. Recent Stanford Primary Achievement, Form W, results were Reading 1.9, Spelling 2.0, and Arithmetic 1.4. Child overactive and distractable."

Medical History

No serious illnesses or injuries.

Mother

Mrs. D. is a slightly obese female who appears her stated age of 28. Her affect fluctuated appropriately with the mood of discussion, but she did not exhibit the normal full range or variation. Her face was almost masklike at times, and she stared blankly on many occasions.

Her general attitude is one of sincere desire to elucidate the dynamics of the problem and if possible to determine methods of improving the situation. Her perception and orientation were normal, and there were no detectable disturbances of reality testing. There was no evidence of bizarre thought processes.

However, the session was quite structured in the sense that the interviewer posed specific questions. Mrs. D. is currently taking Prolixin tablets four times daily, exact dosage unknown.

The MGM is 66 and the MGF is 72,; both living and well. There are seven children in the family, including Mrs. D. Her brother, 35 years old, is the one who now manages the D. family's financial problems and played an active role in having her hospitalized on both occasions. Mrs. D's interaction with the remainder of her siblings is apparently not significant. The mother describes the MGM as kind, loving, and an ideal housewife and mother. The MGM sees Jimmy approximately once a week and apparently has an amiable relationship with him. The MGF is described as intelligent, strong, domineering, and a leader. Mrs. D. states that she was the MGF's favorite child because she appeared to be the most intelligent of the children. MGF is a retired minister. Mrs. D. was an honor student and socially active in high school; she planned to attend college but is vague about why she didn't. She experienced her menarche at the age of 12 years. She was never really taught anything about the physiology of sex at home. She did have dates in high school and appeared to be quite popular. After dating for about 5 months, she and Mr. D. indulged in sexual intercourse, and this was the mother's first sexual experience. She states that her sexual relationships at that time were not satisfactory and have never become so, in that she has never experienced an orgasm. When asked what she liked about the patient's father, she states she was attracted to him physically in "an air force uniform."

According to both parents, the marriage began with a stormy course. The father admittedly had an inferiority complex, and this manifested itself as lack of desire to dominate or manage the home situation and lack of desire to socialize outside the family. The mother states that because of "incompatibility regarding personality" the marriage began with difficulties. The father's introverted personality and inferiority complex persisted in spite of her attempts to persuade him to socialize more actively and to develop a higher self-concept. The mother worked during most of the marriage, including the month before and shortly after Jimmy's birth. Although they openly discussed divorce, they merely continued in their relationship of virtual isolation from one another. Jimmy was cared for by a babysitter during this time. The mother volunteers that she became totally involved in her work and church activities because she "didn't want to go home to the husband I hated." Although this entire period of life is rather vague to the mother now, she states that when Jimmy was 4 years old she felt that she could not live with her husband any longer. She took her son and traveled south to a school for missionaries. She intended to enroll in the school and travel to some foreign country as a missionary. After 5 days, she called her local minister, who reported her location to the family.

They started the proceedings for the mother's first commitment to a mental hospital. She received "intensive psychotherapy and electroshock therapy" for 3 months. Apparently the mother remained relatively stable for the next 2 to 3 years. She again became emotionally upset and began whipping Jimmy with a belt for poor school performance. During this period she also had extramarital relationships on numerous occasions with different men in the community. The father is not aware of this. After a period of approximately 6 months of acting out and the development of manifest symptoms such as distortion of reality testing, Mrs. D. was again hospitalized for 6 weeks. Prior to her most recent hospitalization, sex was the most important thing in her life. Now, however, she feels companionship and social interaction are equally significant. She submits herself to her husband purely as a tool for releasing his sexual drives and overtly ridicules him during his period of excitement shortly before his orgasm. Prior to the mother's most recent acute psychotic episode, she was the manager of financial affairs in the family. At the time of this last hospitalization her brother took over the management of finances and has continued to manage the family finances to the present time.

There has been virtually no interaction between the father and mother or between the mother and Jimmy during the past year. The father has been working the night shift, the mother has been working days, and they see each other during waking hours only about 45 minutes to 1 hour each day. The mother consistently goes to bed at about seven o'clock in the evening, and when the father is at home he and Jimmy sit up alone and watch television. The mother works on Saturday and sleeps most of Sunday.

The mother states that she feels that many of Jimmy's problems are probably manifestations of his disordered family life, and she feels that her two episodes of psychosis and the periods leading up to her hospitalization probably played significant and detrimental roles in his psychologic development. She wants Jimmy to graduate from high school and get a college education. She would like the clinic to elucidate some of the problems contributing to Jimmy's current difficulties and, if possible, give her methods for improving. She is willing to alter her behavior and play an active role to the degree of coming to the clinic regularly, perhaps once a week, if this is what the clinic recommends.

Father

The father is a well-developed, slightly obese male who appears his stated age of 28. He related fairly well with the interviewer. However, there was very poor eye contact. He looked at the floor while he was speaking and displayed mild anxiety when asked direct questions. His verbalizations, on the other hand, were surprisingly lucid. He feels that the problem is directly related to the psychosis of the mother. He has a sincere desire for advice and is willing to modify his behavior, if necessary, to improve the situation.

The PGF is a 55-year-old laborer. He is a chronic alcoholic who was vicious during his drunken stupors and often beat the children and the PGM. The PGPs divorced when the father was 6 years old, and he went to live with his grandparents. During drunken episodes the PGF made fun of the father and of the other children in the areas of personal work and achievement. The father always did poorly in school and did not receive encouragement from the PGF but rather humiliation. This type of repeated negative stimulus nurtured a feeling of inferiority and helped to develop his introverted type of personality. There is very little current interaction between the PGF and the father and no significant contact between the PGF and Jimmy.

The PGM is 52 years old, living and well, and is described by the father as loving, warm, and intelligent. The PGM has successfully entered many writing contests and apparently has been employed as a writer. The father is the oldest of four siblings. He states that his sister and one brother have escaped the humiliation imposed by the PGF and have developed an extrovert type of personality. However, the 16-year-old brother is described by the father as being very much like him, only worse. This brother is extremely shy and avoids social interaction at all costs.

The father always disliked school and did poorly but completed high school. Within the past year or two he has begun to feel he has a greater potential than indicated by is achievements. Therefore, he is learning a new trade as a mold designer. He was engaged to one girl about 1 year before meeting his wife. This engagement did not continue because the girl moved out of state. He had his first sexual experience with his wife about 1 month prior to their marriage and has never had any sexual experiences with other women. The father has been very tolerant of the mother's domineering and often abusive attitude toward him and Jimmy. Recently he has begun to feel his intelligence to be equal to his wife's. This has led to more open clashes with his wife, regarding decisions in family affairs. Except for occasional sexual contact, the father and mother seldom talk or associate with each other.

Four years ago the father suffered a "mild nervous breakdown" manifested by anxiousness and depression. He was treated by a private physician with Stelazine for about 6 months and feels he recovered. He attributes most of Jimmy's problems to the stormy home environment provided by the mother. If he and the mother are divorced he would like to have Jimmy. He has discussed this with the boy, who said he would like to live with his father. Mr. D. desires a diagnosis and counseling from the clinic. He is willing to modify his behavior and be seen in the clinic regularly for some period of time if we so advise. He seems rather pessimistic about the future of his marriage.

Mental Status Examination

Jimmy D. is an 8-year-old boy. He has small features and a crew cut and wears rather thick glasses. He is appropriately dressed in cotton school clothes. He is well oriented. Neuromuscular integration and coordination are good, but there was moderate disturbance in right-left orientation under pressure. He is able to catch and throw a ball vigorously.

Jimmy initially related to the examiner in a teasing manner. He would sit in his chair and smile, giggling occasionally, and would not initiate any spontaneous activity. Later in his play he became active and animated while shooting a dart gun at the blackboard. He fired it at a circular target and at a "monster."

Jimmy told me that he had come to the clinic because he didn't have any friends at school and that most of his play in his neighborhood is with four neighborhood boys: Eddie, age 7; Allen, age 10; Robbie, age 6; and Jerry, age 11. He said that of the four he liked Allen, the 10-year-old, best because he and Allen like to play astronaut and climb trees, playing that they are in spaceships. He said that he did not like Robbie, the 6-year-old, because he is too little and "can't talk right."

Jimmy's fantasy life concerned monsters, being eaten up by monsters, being taken away at night by a burglar, being taken to the burglar's house and then killed, being burned to death, and falling in a sewer. He tells of a "funny dream" wherein he dreamed that he fell into a sewer while trying to get a ball. While in the sewer, he told his friend Robbie to go get—at this point he made a slip and said "my mother," quickly changing it to "my father." "He came and called the police. They came and got me out. We went into the house and watched TV and then I went to sleep. Then I woke up and dreamed that I saw penguins walking into my room, and they laughed at me for sleeping."

In the Raven's Controlled Projection Test, Jimmy told of a 10-year-old boy, named Allen, who liked to play astronaut. Allen's mother and father got angry at him because he got into the trash cans and scattered the trash all over the yard. Allen got mad because his parents were angry. He ran away to Jimmy's house. Allen was especially mad because his parents went after him. Allen's secret was that he had a cat that he was hiding from his mom and dad because his mom and dad wouldn't let him keep it. He took his friends to the cat and they played with it. Allen used to tell stories about going up into space. He told his friends that he has been up into space. This was not true, but he wanted his friends to think so. He told his mother and father that he was sick. He was not sick, but he told them this so he would not have to go to school. Allen was very scared and frightened because the dog bit him. After Allen went to bed he thought about a monster. He was afraid that the monster would get him. When he fell asleep he dreamed that the monster did get him and that the monster ate him. He woke up because he was so frightened of the monster. Allen's three wishes were for a space capsule, a kitty cat, and a space suit, and if Allen had a lot of money he would buy a box of toys. Allen also wanted to be a dog because a dog can bite. Jimmy said that he liked the story because Allen was very much like him. They both liked astronauts. Allen was different from him because Allen ran away from home and had a kitty cat.

Jimmy said that he had trouble making friends because they like to start fights and they don't like him because he failed the first grade. He likes to play with boys because girls like to play house. He has been sleeping with his mother almost every night up until last week when his dad got a new job. At night he fears that a man, a burglar, will come and steal him and take him away and kill him. If he saw a burglar he would "holler and tell his dad to get his gun."

Jimmy was afraid to come to the child psychiatry clinic because he feared that I would put a stick down his throat and he would choke. He said, "I worry about dying a lot. I worry that it would hurt. I wouldn't like it." He said that he first started worrying about dying when his family moved 3 years ago. An attic of a barbershop burned across the street from their house, and he began to worry that he might catch fire, burn up, and die. If he died he wouldn't get to see anybody anymore. He said that he didn't like their town because it has too many people and they are always having fires. He wishes he could move where Grandma and Grandpa live.

His mother and father fight about "little things" like "if Daddy leaves a sock around, Mommy gets mad at him. One time Mommy hit Daddy over the head with a toy gun and broke it. Mommy also gets mad at Daddy because Daddy won't help her bring in the groceries." His favorite parent is his father. He enjoys taking company trips with his father. His mother was a patient in the hospital. "When Mommy was sick she ran away from home with me and we went to Georgia." I asked how his mother acts while sick and he replied, "She gets mean; she acts mean." Jimmy said, "I would like to have an older brother and sister. They could play with me when I don't have no friends. My dad plays with me. We wrestle once in a while but not often enough. I keep trying to get him to and he won't. He's too busy watching TV. I like *The Green Hornet* because they fight and stuff. Mommy likes to go to bed every night at seven-thirty. Daddy and I watch television together."

When asked to draw a picture, Jimmy drew first a house, saying that he could draw a house better than anything else. He then drew a figure with a smiling face standing in front of the house. When I asked him to draw his family, he drew his father to the extreme left and labeled it Harold. Jimmy drew his mother in the center, labeling it Sylvia, and drew himself at the right, labeling it Jimmy. The father and Jimmy look exactly alike except that the father is taller and Jimmy has bigger feet. All figures have a smiling face and all are complete.

Jimmy particularly enjoyed playing pass with me with the basketball and became very friendly toward me as we were doing this. Regarding his problems, he said that he wished the other kids liked him better and that he didn't have to worry about dying. He does not think that he has any serious problems with his studies or with his parents.

Psychologic Testing

Procedures Used

    Wechsler Intelligence Scale for Children (partial)
    Bender
    Visual Motor Gestalt Test

Jimmy, age 8-3, was tested primarily to obtain a basic estimate of his intellectual capacity. The complete WISC was not given. Prorated IQ estimates were based on the information, comprehension, vocabulary, picture completion, block design, and coding subtests. The results obtained yielded a verbal IQ of 103, performance IQ of 82, and full-scale IQ of 92. The test results suggest a child who is somewhat impulsive in interpersonal relationships and often confused by the demands of academic tasks. It is the examiner's impression that a high level of anxiety and short attention are interfering with his academic achievement, but a trial of therapy or further projective testing would be necessary to confirm this impression.

Diagnostic Conference Formulation

Jimmy is an 8-year-old male whose poor academic performance and difficulties in forming satisfactory peer relationships seem to have resulted from the chronic emotional turmoil in his home. He has experienced parental ambivalence and confusion about aggression, sex, male-female roles, and child-adult relations. He may be closely identified with his passive underachieving father. His poor attention to schoolwork is probably the result of preoccupation in fantasy with the aggression that he sees everywhere. Pretending everyone is happy, moving to the grandparents, and having siblings are all fantasied solutions for lessening his fears. In spite of many traumatic emotional experiences, Jimmy has adequate reality contact and still desires interhuman relations.

Mrs. D. has had two hospitalizations for acute psychotic reactions. She has intellectual understanding of her problems with her husband and child. However, her capacity for empathic human relations is limited. Although she functions satisfactorily in her work, her hold on reality is tenuous and she appears unable to find personal gratification in either the mother or wife role.

Mr. D. has a poor self-concept and has always been an underachiever. Since his wife's illnesses became so acute he has begun to question his inferiority to her. Even so, he is afraid or, for other reasons, is only marginally able to cope with her aggression or to manage the financial and other affairs of family living. At present he desires to improve things but is unable to help either himself or Jimmy.

DSM III Diagnosis

Axis I. 309.24—Adjustment disorder with anxious mood
309.23—Adjustment disorder with academic inhibition
Axis II. V71.09—Unable to establish a diagnosis of a specific learning disorder
Axis III. No physical illness
Axis IV. Stress: 5; Severe; chronic recurring mental illness in the mother and harsh parental discipline
Axis V. Highest adaptive functioning in past year; 6; failed first grade and poor peer relationships

Staff Recommendations

1. Individual psychotherapy for Jimmy. We will try to offer him male identification, an opportunity to ventilate his fears, and help in understanding his world.
2. Unless Jimmy's environment can be improved, his therapy will not be effective. It may be necessary to place him out of the home, but first, intensive counseling with the parents should be tried.

Mr. D. will be seen weekly by a therapist to help him achieve a better appraisal of his abilities, to encourage him to assume a stronger role in managing family affairs, and to help him find ways of protecting Jimmy from Mrs. D.'s irrational outbursts and erratic behavior.

With concurrence of the referring physician, we will assume the management of Mrs. D.'s medication. (It is usually more efficient for the clinic to assume the responsibility for the mental health care of the entire family, but we are careful not to do so without full agreement from the referring physician and the family member.) She is not at this point a candidate for insight psychotherapy. Rather, we will try to capitalize upon her intellectual ability to help her accept more decisive behavior from the father and to suppress her impulsive and aggressive behavior.

Follow-up Treatment Summary

The reader will be interested to know that this family accepted the treatment recommendations of the staff. Initially, Jimmy was very frightened, jittery, and evasive in his therapy sessions. However, after a few weeks he indulged in fantasy play and direct discussion of his family and school problems. He changed from being overtly aggressive with peers to being submissive and a scapegoat. More recently, he formed a few normal give-and-take friendships. The school reported marked improvement, and with considerable effort Jimmy passed to the next grade.

The mother attended clinic regularly. At one point she became increasingly delusional in her thinking and conversations. As a result she lost her job, but another hospitalization was averted by adjustment of her medication. She stopped sleeping with Jimmy and leaves his discipline to the father. She remains overtly hostile to the father but moved with him to a house nearer his work and away from her relatives under his threat of leaving.

Mr. D. progressed in his new job and did satisfactorily in night school. He remains very shy and uncertain, seeking much advice and reassurance. At present he is uncertain whether or not to continue the marriage. He has taken the financial responsibilities from his brother-in-law and no longer discusses his marital problems with Jimmy. He accepts the responsibility for the child's discipline.

Eventually, Jimmy became relatively anxiety-free and was able to do average work in school. His nightmares abated, and he seemed to develop some understanding of his mother's illness. Regular therapy sessions for Jimmy and his father were discontinued. Medication-free trials for the mother showed that she simply could not go without medication for long periods. On maintenance dosage, she is able to work and does not get so upset with Jimmy's behavior. She is not happy but accepts her realistic dependency on the father. Jimmy remains "at risk" for adjustment problems. As too often happens the clinic has lost contact with this family. We hope they will seek professional assistance as needed.

SUMMARY

The case study method has been illustrated by three cases presented in detailed summary form, following the outline presented early in this chapter. This outline offers a structure for recording examination data and facilitates the diagnostic and treatment formulation when single, specific etiology of symptoms cannot be identified.

The first case illustrated a child's and mother's reaction to an acute emotional stress. The second boy illustrates the result of a combination of untoward sociocultural experiences and an emotionally stressful mother–child interaction pattern. In the third instance we have reviewed a boy whose school performance was considerably below his native ability because of the chronic stress of living with psychologically ill parents. However, Jimmy's school symptoms could not be considered merely "a reaction" to an untoward environment in the sense that he would begin to perform adequately if he were removed from the home or if the marital maladjustment were resolved. There was evidence of disturbances within the boy himself as manifested by his poor object relationships, his continuous concern over aggression and violence in himself and others about him, his psychic discomfort (about which he readily told the examiner), his excessive reliance on fantasy to cope with anxiety, and a concomitant lessening of actual creative or productive activities in school and in play.

Treatment of Jeffrey, the boy having school phobia, was primarily aimed at relieving his conflicts over the loss of his grandmother with no direct explanation or interpretation of his neurotically close identification with his mother. Treatment of the mother's depression and her acceptance of Jeff's striving for independence seemed to be sufficient to permit the child's resumption of normal school performance.

Granville's treatment was not simple, since the formation of adequate self-identity, social concepts, and impulse control seemed seriously impaired. Initially, treatment focused on supplying some of the social deficiencies of his environment and attenuating his anger by better dependency gratification. His mother needed to be helped to find a more gratifying life before she could begin to help her son toward a socially desirable maturation.

Jimmy D., the last case example, illustrates the need for treatment of multiple members of the family at whatever level each can effectively use. The D. family exemplifies a situation rather frequently seen among our clinic families in that the psychologically most disturbed member is permitted to dictate the most important family decisions. Although the chronicity of the parents' difficulties makes one cautious about the ultimate prognosis, there is every hope that the untoward effect of the parent's adjustment was minimized for Jimmy.

10

TREATMENT PLANNING

As noted in Chapter 1, treatment of emotional and behavior problems in children from the time of Hippocrates (460 B.C.) has consisted primarily of instructing or admonishing parents. This remained the modus operandi of physicians well into the so-called Child Guidance Movement of this century. Even Freud,[13] in the first decade of the 20th century, had only one brief conversation with little Hans. The treatment of Hans's phobia was carried out by the father under Freud's instructions. Reports of direct psychoanalysis of children did appear in the literature. However, most clinicians saw children for evaluation only and not for direct psychotherapy until the 1940s. Treatment consisted of giving advice to the parents, to the court or to the child's school. During and immediately after World War II, individual psychotherapy for children came into practice.[16] For a variety of theoretical and pragmatic reasons most children did not receive classic psychoanalytic therapy, but much of their psychotherapy was based upon psychoanalytic and neo-analytic precepts. Since that time, many varieties or variations of psychotherapy and other treatment methods have come into use.

THE RELATION OF DIAGNOSIS TO TREATMENT

It is beyond the scope of this text to give an in-depth dissertation on all of the different kinds of psychiatric treatments available. Such a treatise would require a consensual definition of each treatment, the technical skills and knowledge necessary for its use, its indications and contraindications, its efficacy and cost-effectiveness. The resulting dissertation would fill several volumes and require multiple authors. Only recently have we begun to develop the methodologies that will permit us to make objective, scientific analyses of our treatment methods.

We can, however, discuss "treatment planning" or the selection of treatment(s) most likely to help a given child and family. Such treatment plans can be based upon the existing concepts about psychopathology and the pathogenesis of various symptoms and symptom clusters. Rosenzweig[20] laments that *DSM III* "completely avoids concepts of psychopathology." The manual has greatly improved the reliability of psychiatric diagnosis by its descriptive nature and its multiaxial format, but this reliability has been achieved perhaps at "considerable expense to validity." *DSM III* is no doubt good for research purposes, but it is much less useful in everyday clinical practice. Resembling a "cookbook," its format requires relatively little clinical skill for use. In his APA presidential address Langsley[17] insists, "There is no substitute for clinical skills." Clinical skills are too abstract and subjective to be taught by the printed word alone. Most conscientious readers will spend the rest of their professional lives learning and refining clinical skills. It is this fact that makes individual supervision so essential for the training of young professionals and for learning about therapy.

We have learned rather quickly that *DSM III* describes and classifies mental disorders, not mental illnesses. In fact, the *DSM III* Committee was unable to define "mental illness." It is unrealistic at this point to expect any nosological system to give us much guidance in treatment. The system tells us a great deal about our own and our colleagues' patients, but it does not provide treatment guides. The five-axial diagnosis does hint at psychopathology and may imply cause(s), but in each case with considerable uncertainty. Diagnosis still lacks the information needed to lead us directly to treatment.

A RATIONALE FOR TREATMENT PLANNING

The history of medicine shows that many times effective treatments have been empirically discovered long before specific causes were known. The convulsive disorders, diabetes and the leukemias are notable examples. Psychotropic medications and the psychotherapies relieve much suffering in conditions of uncertain etiology. It is even reasonable to believe that research into treatment can lead us toward greater understanding of pathology and etiology although ideally we might wish to know the cause(s) before we select the treatments.

Until future knowledge dictates otherwise I propose to use the designation "treatment planning" rather than the term "treatment." The therapeutic plan is based upon the full case study and the "diagnostic formulation" rather than on the "diagnosis" or diagnostic classification. The treatment plan must be aimed at alleviating the development, psychic, academic and social (including family) problems of the child. These "problems" must actually exist and be clearly defined. For example, a child who consistently scores below average on the nationally standardized achievement tests has a learning problem reflecting an intellectual impairment, a specific learning disability, or an emotional illness that interferes with learning. On the other hand, if the presenting complaint is "not living up to potential in school" there may or may not be a learning problem. In the first instance, the child is compared with national achievement scores. In the second instance, he/she may be at the national "norm" but not living up to parental hopes or expectations. In this latter situation there probably is a parent-child problem, but it may be more complicated than that.

The origins, pathogenesis and prognosis of the problems must be comprehended as much as possible. The treatment methods chosen must have some hope of relieving the identified problem(s) and be skillfully applied and carefully monitored. The word *problem* is used here in the generic sense to include all of the questions listed under "Diagnostic Formulation" presented in Chapter 7. The complete case study should supply the answers to the following questions:

1. How sick or impaired is this child?
2. In which areas of functioning is the impairment manifested, and in what areas does he/she function well?
3. Is there any past or present evidence that the central nervous system is not functionally intact?
4. Which psychosocial factors in the past life probably contributed to the problem(s)?
5. Which psychosocial factors in the current life continue to contribute to the problem(s) or are likely to be an impediment to recovery?
6. Which of the factors considered in questions 2, 3, 4 and 5 must be changed to allow improvement to occur?

7. Which additional factors ought to be changed for the child's general well-being although perhaps not directly related to the presenting problems?
8. Which methods, if any, can be used to effect the desired changes?

IMPORTANT ELEMENTS OF THE DIAGNOSTIC FORMULATION

Using both direct observation and history from parents and teachers, we gain an overall impression of the extent of social, developmental and mental impairment the child has in comparison with peers and with society's ideal. We use the items of the mental status examination outlined in Chapter 4 to record the areas of good functioning and of poor functioning. We consider these items to be either ego functions or reflections upon one or more ego functions. For example, K. C., the 13½-month-old boy cited in Chapter 6, functioned well in every area compared to his age group. We could find no areas of impairment or potentially harmful environmental situations. The only reason K. C. was examined by a psychiatrist was that he was a burn victim and was included in a research project. No psychiatric treatment was indicated or offered. Psychiatric clinicians have dilemmas in deciding whether or not to offer therapy. Not every child brought to us needs it.

Contrast K. C. with Bobbie M., 42 months old, also reported in Chapter 6. Bobbie was very difficult to examine and had to be seen several times to develop an accurate mental status evaluation. He showed impairment or was suspected of impairment in every one of the items on the mental status outline. His mental picture did change over the ensuing 4 or 5 years. We came to know that he had no problems with orientation and his perceptual apparatus was intact. He was not mentally retarded and did not have a specific learning disability. No definite central nervous system abnormalities were demonstrated by clinical or laboratory examinations or by neuropsychologic testing, but after 3 years of therapy, his clinicians still wondered whether his brain were physiologically normal. (Scientists have yet to prove that "minimal brain dysfunction" really exists.) Projective testing did not demonstrate a formal thought disorder in Bobbie, but his current and previous therapists had serious questions about that also. On all of the other mental status items

Bobbie showed mild to very serious impairments at different times. He demonstrated ability to make meaningful relationships with adults (mother, teachers and therapists), but he was often immature and clinging and his interactions revealed extremes of ambivalence. There was never any doubt about Bobbie's need for treatment, but several staff questioned whether or not it would have to be in a residential or hospital setting. Additional rationales for selecting specific treatments will be discussed later in this chapter within the context of the entire diagnostic formulation.

We have responded to the first three questions of the diagnostic formulation for K. C. and for Bobbie. With respect to past and present psychosocial stressors (questions 4 and 5) there were none for K. C., but many for Bobbie. Bobbie is a twin. Although birth weight was near normal and early development was reported within the normal range, statistically, one or both twins are more at risk for developmental or emotional disorders than single births. His mother was living at a marginal economic level with three small children. She had a rather chaotic marriage that ended in divorce. Her own adolescence was stormy, and she continued in psychological warfare with her own mother. Intermittently, she suffered depressions for which she had steadfastly refused treatment. She seemed quite ineffective in providing a home structure and firm behavioral limits for her children. She had much trouble admitting that Bobbie was disturbed and brought him to the clinic under much pressure from her welfare worker. Obviously, there were many factors in Bobbie and his mother that urgently needed attention. Selecting treatment methods that would be effective remained a constant problem and often shook the therapists' confidence in themselves.

THE AVAILABLE TREATMENT METHODS

What treatments do we have for the children who have many problems who are brought to us? Long-term-outcome studies have consistently failed to demonstrate that one method of psychotherapy of the various disorders is significantly more effective than another or better than placebos or no treatment. Most of these studies were in the 1960s and were retrospective. These confusing findings are hardly surprising when one considers the tremendous number of possible etiologic variables and the relationships and interdigitations of these variables with each other contributing to the clinical picture. In addition to the severity of the ego impairments in the child and the past and present stressors within the environment, the chronicity of the problem(s) may be crucial to outcome. A developmental regression from any cause can become a new stress and thereby serve as a cause of additional psychopathology.[11] Additional variables that must be kept in mind when planning treatment are the child's age and physical health, the cultural and social milieu, genetic endowment, a possible innate maturational timetable and the biases or blind spots of the clinician(s) in charge.

Concerned about the lack of demonstrable differences in the effectiveness of various "schools" of psychotherapy, Truax[24,25] studied some personality attributes of therapists. He found that those rated high in empathy, genuineness and warmth had a significantly higher improvement rate than therapists rated low in these characteristics. Without controlling for the therapists' personality the large-scale studies of the 1960s tended to show a 65 to 85 per cent improvement rate irrespective of the theoretical tenets of the therapists. Another factor affecting outcome may be selection of the wrong treatment for the pathology at hand.

With the present state of our knowledge, therapists must be aware of the grave responsibilities they have and hope for future research that will enhance our clinical skills and answer our questions. One cannot be a therapeutic nihilist and still help children. At the same time our motto must be *primum non nocere.* We know that the possibility of success in helping the child is much better than chance if we use therapeutic technics that we know and understand well and in which we have confidence. However, we must be thoroughly familiar with as many types of treatment as we can, use careful judgment in choosing them and be prepared to try something else if the child's condition worsens or fails to improve. Because of the child's social, biologic and psychologic dependency we should always try to involve his adult caretakers in active, constructive participation in the therapy.[21] The following is a brief review of some of the commonly used treatment methods, with a few comments and references.

FAMILY COUNSELING

Counseling parents (child guidance) and environmental manipulations are two of the oldest and most widely used forms of treatment used to help children with developmental deviations or emotional problems. Counseling parents can be very effective for treating the transient situational reactions or adjustment disorders that result from the stress of death, divorce or battles over custody and visitation, and for some phobias, habit disturbances, sleep problems, eating disorders, and sleep terrors in very young children. Two frequent problems inherent in parental counseling are that some therapists do not realize the value of involving both parents in the counseling and that when good results are not obtained, the therapist may dismiss the family rather than search for more serious psychopathology or try another treatment approach. Simple guidance often works well with acute problems but is less likely to be effective in chronic situations.

Under the topic "environmental manipulations" we include changing neighborhoods or schools, foster placements, group homes, residential treatment placement, hospitalization and referrals for care by the juvenile justice system. These manipulations are often tried with or without professional advice. Sometimes such maneuvers have been helpful to the child. However, blind, capricious placement of children can have many far-reaching consequences and except in emergencies should not be done without first carefully evaluating the child and family. A 1986 issue of *Newsweek*[15] reported that the psychiatric hospitalization of persons 18 years old and younger doubled between 1970 and 1980 and increased 350 per cent in 1980–84. They cite possible reasons for this growth of admissions, including increased availability of beds, better insurance coverage, and decriminalization of "status offenses." They quote some sources as questioning whether many of these hospitalizations are "really necessary." They also quote several clinicians who believe that most parents turn to the psychiatrist in desperation as a "last resort." The current availability of immediate psychiatric treatment for minors is long overdue and is certainly welcomed by most mental health professionals. If some "unnecessary" hospitalizations are occurring we should be able to correct that with a few years of experience and with some improvements in our alternative (outpatient) treatment facilities and financing. In the past, psychiatric hospitalization has often been looked upon as an end in itself rather than a means to an end. These new hospital facilities must not become "warehouses" for the "storage" of children with bad prognoses.

The return to such an archaic situation can be prevented if we carefully monitor each patient's progress and offer first-rate continuity of care. Fortunately, the high cost of treatment in these new facilities will probably prevent us from doing otherwise. Children with truly treatment-refractory disorders have to receive continued care in an environment that is "least restrictive" yet reasonable in cost and duly concerned for personal and public safety.

Marriage and divorce counseling[22,23] are offered by child psychiatric clinics as well as many other professionals. Child clinicians tend to focus on relieving the stress on the children in the family. Other professionals no doubt have concern for the entire family but are likely to focus primarily on the marriage and the partners. Caution must be observed if we offer only marriage therapy as an indirect way of helping a child. If the child has symptoms of any consequence, treating his/her stressors (the parents) may simply not effect a cure. We may wonder that only one child in a dysfunctional family suffers symptoms. We do not understand why our patient's siblings seem to do so well while living in the same chaotic family. Clinicians must always look for contributing factors within the symptomatic child himself or for family "scapegoating."

PSYCHOTHERAPY

Individual psychotherapy[1,5,6,9] for the child or for the child and one or both parents is still widely used. In the past there has been much effort to differentiate "supportive" psychotherapy from "insight-oriented" psychotherapy, but such distinctions are becoming less important. When one has the rare opportunity of a detailed review of individual psychotherapy hour by hour, it seems that most psychotherapists are becoming more and more eclectic and that they will use whatever approach they feel will be helpful at a given time. Discussions of differences in psychotherapeutic approaches now seem to be academic exercises in semantics that do not really reflect the daily interchanges in our consultation rooms. It certainly makes sense empirically that in most cases we must support our patients as well as strive for insight. Adams[1] states that analytically oriented therapy is not at all incompatible with supportive therapy or with behavior therapy technics. In reading and listening to him, one does not receive the impression that he is blindly wedded to any "theoretical school." He is very child- and family-oriented, tunes in to his patients with all of his perceptual senses, and tries to comprehend and offers help according to the patient's needs and abilities rather than by "the school's" dictum.

Why do so many clinicians still use psychotherapy after 45 years of experience with no support of its effectiveness from the many "outcome studies"? The answer may be that psycho- therapists know that such studies are full of methodologic flaws. Therapists know that psychotherapy does help, although often not as much or as quickly or as efficiently as we would wish. It should also be noted that many, perhaps most, psy- chotherapists are now offering their therapy along with one or more of the other treatment modalities reviewed in this chapter. Perhaps the multiaxial diagnostic system has helped us see the need for more than one treatment modality in most cases.

Psychoanalysis had to undergo many changes to accommo- date to children.[10-12] Although analytically oriented psycho- therapy is widely used, classical psychoanalysis of children has not been practiced extensively in much of Europe and in the midwestern United States. There may be many social and economic reasons for this. Like most other psychotherapies, analysis often helps youth who have been refractory to other methods. Its indications and cost-effectiveness are still prob- lematic. From personal communications and informal obser- vations it appears that psychoanalysts have also become more eclectic in their practices.

BEHAVIOR MODIFICATION

Behavior therapy is considered by some to be a form of "sup- portive" psychotherapy, yet it is quite different in being very action-oriented and goal-directed. Insight can and does develop during the course of behavioral therapy, but this is incidental and not a primary requisite. Some early authors such as Ferster[8] denied the existence or the relevance of the unconscious; how- ever, such arguments have become passé. Behavior therapy may in some instances be the technic of choice for crisis interven- tion, brief therapy and behavior alteration, and it can be either the major therapeutic mode or an adjunct in the management of many psychiatric disorders.[3] The use of this treatment by persons who are not knowledgeable about the principles of operant conditioning and behavior therapy or are careless or incompetent in its application does not help the child and may produce adverse reactions. To be effective, behavior therapy requires considerable cooperation, understanding and mutual trust among the adults in the child's home, school or hospital milieu. Unlike Pavlov's reflex conditioning of dogs, operant conditioning requires that the "stimulus" (reward) follows the response and that the reward must have positive value for the child. Without constant monitoring, a behavior modification plan can deteriorate into crass bribery or a coercive manipulation game between the child and his adults. When such deterioration occurs, the therapy fails or at the least has no long-term effect upon the child.

GROUP THERAPY

Group therapy also has been used to provide support, to produce insight and to effect social training. It seems to be especially beneficial for children and adolescents in the hospital wards. In the outpatient situation the clinician must be affiliated with a clinic or have a very large practice in order to use group therapy in a cost-effective way. Comparatively few clinicians use this as the sole form of therapy, although its use at specific times during a long therapeutic course can be very beneficial for the child.

FAMILY GROUP THERAPY

Recently, learning family group therapy has become a requirement of training for all psychiatric residents in the United States.[23] It behooves all child psychiatry clinicians to become knowledgeable about family dynamics and to learn how to use family group therapy.[4] I have used it in my practice both as a primary method of therapy and as an adjunct with traditional individual psychotherapy. It is not a panacea but is often dramatically helpful, and there are exciting possibilities for future research that may help with many of the technical problems associated with treating families (see Chapter 2).

HYPNOTHERAPY

In a tertiary care pediatric hospital my colleagues and I find hypnotherapy and relaxation therapy especially helpful in reducing pain, fear, uncooperativeness and excessive need for narcotics associated with life-threatening illnesses and tedious, sometimes painful medical procedures. Most children are easily hypnotized and they really respond to the sense of mastery and control they can have with hypnosis and self-hypnosis. Gardner and Olness[14] give an excellent review of the technics and the many uses for hypnosis.

PSYCHOPHARMACOTHERAPY

Psychopharmacotherapy has been studied and used with children since the introduction of anticonvulsants and stimulants in the mid-1930s.[27,28] Clinical use of psychotropic medications and research into their indications and contraindications have been extremely slow to get under way. Lack of trained staff, humanistic and legal concerns and seemingly insurmountable methodologic problems have all blocked progress. Just now, in the current decade, we do see some hope of conquering research design and methodologic impediments to progress.[27]

Much of the current research regarding drugs of choice for specific mental disorders remains inconclusive. However, there is growing evidence of their usefulness in the management of specific target symptoms. It is strongly recommended that psychotropic medication be combined with one or more of the other forms of therapy. The family or the child's guardians must always be involved in the treatment. Regarding the major tranquilizers and the antidepressants,[19] research is inconclusive, but there is empiric evidence that children may receive enough relief from their primary emotional distresses to resume learning at school and benefit from social training at home. Sometimes such relief is a prerequisite for the child's participation in his own psychotherapy. When children are suffering significant psychic stress, relieving them with medication not only is humane but often does much to promote a relationship in which insight-oriented psychotherapy can occur. However, medications can make the child excessively dependent on the therapist. Some clinicians fear that relieving the child's psychic distress may lessen the motivation for working on problems. These issues are not indications for or contraindications against medication, rather, they are factors that must be considered with the child and family within the context of the patient-therapist relationship.

In treating Attention Deficit Disorders[7] the stimulants seem to help the hyperactivity and attention problems but have little direct effect on the associated learning disabilities or behavior problems. The child may need remedial education and behavior therapy in addition to the stimulant medication. Effective dosage levels also are very important and must be individually adjusted. In many cases that are referred to us because the stimulants "didn't work," we find that dosages were inadequate and that too little attention was given to the child's learning disorders, dissocial behavior patterns and family turmoil. There is still no conclusive evidence that the benzodiazepines, antihistamines or other drugs often used to treat the anxiety disorders act more quickly or more effectively than psychotherapy alone.[26] However, one may be professionally obligated for the sake of the child to try these drugs when psychotherapy and parental counseling are not sufficiently helpful.

There can be an ethical and professional dilemma created when one or both parents refuse psychotherapy but want medicine with which to control, perhaps manipulate, the child's behavior. If the child or family is in great stress I am willing to prescribe medication. If the desire for medication is mainly a resistance to looking at the need for change in others besides the child, I still may prescribe, but see them frequently for short appointments to try to make a trusting relationship that can eventually lead to changes in the family. Sometimes, if just one member of the family changes, the others follow. Very often, though, dysfunctional families are quite refractory to change, and the psychologically most unstable one among them is given or permitted to have the dominant or decision-making role.

EDUCATIONAL THERAPY

Remedial education and various types of social training are widely available in the schools and other community agencies. The overall effectiveness of these measures is unknown, but many of these agencies seek psychiatric consultation for selected children, hoping to find other or additional treatments.

For many of such referred children medication and/or family therapy is needed in addition to remedial education.

The reader is encouraged to reread the follow-up treatment of Bobbie M. in Chapter 6. He may not be typical of psychiatric clinic patients. However, the case illustrates the multiple nature and complexity of the problems presented by some children and the flexibility and tenacity often required of therapists.

Child therapists who know only one form of treatment have limited social usefulness. Many different strategies are necessary for helping a child and his family, and these needs should be evident from our diagnostic formulations and the treatment reviews of our cases.

SUMMARY

Psychiatric treatment of child and adolescent mental disorders has become increasingly complex but, it is hoped, more effective. It takes more than a kind heart and good intentions to give many of these young people real help. We can no longer subscribe to the concept of "one diagnosis and one treatment."

Lack of knowledge about etiology is a stumbling block, but not an insurmountable one. I offer a treatment-planning approach based on generally accepted concepts about psychopathology and pathogenesis. A plan for a specific child requires careful evaluation of the child and the environment along with knowledgeable selection of treatment methods. The child's adults must be actively involved in the treatment. On the basis of careful regular monitoring of progress, changes of treatment methods or even changes of therapists must be considered from time to time. To prevent budget makers and third-party payors from making treatment decisions, all therapists must have constant concern for cost-effectiveness.

I have sometimes been grateful that an apparent innate maturational timetable within the child and even time itself seem to assist in the child's recovery. Yet we cannot depend upon such intangibles. Improved research[18] into causes of illness and treatment methods is urgently needed. We also must find ways to identify truly treatment-refractory children objectively and to provide for their continued humane care.

REFERENCES

1. Adams, Paul: *A Primer of Child Psychotherapy.* Little, Brown & Co., Boston, 2d Ed., 1982.
2. American Psychiatric Association: *Diagnostic and Statistical Manual of Mental Disorders (DSM III).* 3d Ed., Washington, D.C., 1980.
3. Birk, L. & Bird, A.B.: The learning therapies, in *Overview of the Psychotherapies,* G. Usdin (Ed.). New York, Brunner/Mazel, 1975, pp. 51–68.
4. Brown, S.L.: *Diagnosis, clinical management and family interviewing in childhood and adolescence, in Science and Psychoanalysis,* Vol. 14. M.S. Wasserman, (Ed.). New York, Grune and Stratton, 1969, pp. 188–198.
5. Chessick, R.D.: *Techniques and Practice of Intensive Psychotherapy.* New York, Jason Aronson, Inc., 1974.
6. Cooper, S. and Wanerman, L.: *Children in Treatment: A Primer for Beginning Psychotherapists.* New York, Brunner/Mazel, 1977.
7. Donnelly, M. and Rapoport, J.L.: *Attention Deficit Disorders in Diagnosis and Psychopharmacology of Childhood and Adolescent Disorders,* J.M. Wiener (Ed.). New York, John Wiley & Son, 1985, pp. 179–189.
8. Ferster, C.B.: *The Experimental Analysis of Human Behavior and the Environmental Control, in An Introduction to the Science of Human Behavior* by J.I. Nurnberger et al. New York, Appleton-Century-Crofts, 1963, pp. 199–239.
9. Frank, J.D.: *An Overview of Psychotherapy,* Chapter 1 in *Overview of the Psychotherapies,* G. Usdin (Ed.). New York, Brunner/Mazel, 1975, pp. 3–25.
10. Freud, A.: *The Psychoanalytic Treatment of Children.* London, Imago Publishing Co., 1946.
11. ———: Regression as a principle in mental development. Menninger Clin. Bull., *27*:126, 1963.
12. ———: *Normality and Pathology in Childhood.* New York, International Universities Press, 1965, pp. 54–140.
13. Freud, S.: Analysis of a phobia in a five-year-old boy (1909), in *Collected Papers,* Vol. II, translated by Alix and James Strachey. London, Hogarth Press, 1949, pp. 149–288.
14. Gardner, J. and Olness, K.: *Hypnosis and Hypnotherapy with Children.* New York, Grune and Stratton, Inc., 1981.
15. Gelman, D., Raine, G., Jackson, J.T., Katz, S., Weathers, D., and Copolla, V.: Treating teens in trouble: Can the psychiatric ward fill in for the family? Newsweek, January 20, 1986, pp. 52–54.
16. Haworth, M. (Ed.): *Child Psychotherapy.* New York, Basic Books, 1964.
17. Langsley, D.G.: Presidential address: Today's teachers and tomorrow's psychiatrists. Am. J. Psychiatry, *138*:1013–1016, 1981.
18. Phillips, I., Cohen, R., and Enzer, N. (eds): *The Future of Child Psychiatry.* Washington, D.C., American Academy of Child Psychiatry, 1983.
19. Ping-Antich, J., Ryan, N.D., Rabinovich, H.: Affective disorders in childhood and adolescence, in *Diagnosis and Psychopharmacology of Childhood and Adolescent Disorders,* J.M. Wiener (Ed.). New York, John Wiley & Sons, 1985.
20. Rosenzweig, N.: Diagnosis and the concept of mental illness. Am. J. Soc. Psychiatry, *II*:47–50, 1982.
21. Simmons, J.E.: Parent treatability: What is it? J. Am. Acad. Child Psychiatry, *20*:4, 1981.
22. Steinzor, B.: *When Parents Divorce.* New York, Pantheon Books, 1969.
23. Sugarman, S.: Family therapy training in psychiatric education. J. Psychiatr. Educ., *9*:148–155, 1985.
24. Truax, C.B.: Therapist empathy, genuineness and warmth and patient therapeutic outcome. J. Consult. Psychol., *30*:395–401, 1966.

25. Truax, C.B. and Carkhuff, R.R.: *Toward Effective Counseling and Psychotherapy.* Chicago, Aldine Publishing Company, 1967.
26. White, J.H.: *Pediatric Psychopharmacology.* Baltimore, Williams & Wilkins, Co., 1977.
27. Wiener, J.M., Ed.: *Diagnosis and Psychopharmacology of Childhood and Adolescent Disorders.* New York, John Wiley & Sons, 1985.
28. ——— and Jaffe, S.L.: Historical overview of childhood and adolescent psychopharmacology in *Diagnosis and Psychopharmacology of Childhood and Adolescent Disorders,* J.M. Wiener (Ed.). New York, John Wiley & Sons, 1985.

11

CONSULTATIONS

For many years, Dr. Gerald Caplan[6,7] has written about primary and secondary prevention in psychiatry. He acknowledged the usefulness of the traditional consultant-patient model of consultation. However, for purposes of preventive psychiatry, he endorsed the consultant-consulter or consultant-community model. He stated, "A community focus does not entail neglect of the individual, but rather a wider responsibility." Caplan hoped that through the community the psychiatrist could effect the emotional health not only of identified patients, but of many individuals who are "at risk" but not currently identified. This concept has had special appeal to child psychiatrists who are keenly aware of the very small numbers in their specialty compared with the very large population of youth in our society. We also know that many other professionals (social and child-caring agencies, schools, and so on) have much more direct contact with children than we do, especially during the very important early developmental years. Effective preventive measures can reach more children if they are taught to child care providers and nonpsychiatric medical professionals.

Berlin[5] calls the consultant-consulter model "an indirect method of helping the child." He patterns his work after the approach described by Coleman in 1947. The consultant focuses on the feelings of the consulter to help the latter be more effective with the child. This can often be more beneficial than directly advising the consulter on ways to deal with the patient. Berlin has also reviewed program, administrative and systems consultation using the consultant-consulter model, which differs significantly from the traditional medical model of specific patient consultation.

Wise and Berlin[25] discuss the role of ambiguity, role conflict and other stresses on the consultant. They, along with many other authors,[2,4,12,15,19,20] write about the distaste residents have for consultation work, the stress and "burnout" of consultants and the feelings of despair some have about our relationship with pediatrics. On the surface it may seem that our effectiveness and personal satisfactions would be greater in working with nonmedical colleagues. However, Roeske[18] does not paint such a rosy picture. "We (child psychiatrists), through the child guidance movement from 1909, were creative leaders in comprehensive care and the team concept." Others do not credit child psychiatry with these innovations, and now in the last quarter of this century we find ourselves "on the fringe of the changing health care delivery system."[18] Child psychiatry seems to overlap with every field and has no identified unique social usefulness. The theme that emanates from these concerned authors is that the consultant-consuler model produces the greatest frustration for the child psychiatric consultant. Although the consultant-patient model produces less emotional stress, the heavy service load can be exhausting. With this latter model, teaching opportunities are limited and the potential for primary prevention, a philosophy dear to our hearts, is practically nil.

LEARNING CONSULTATION SKILLS

With so much "doom and gloom" in the literature I hesitated to include a chapter on consultation in a book written for the beginner child psychiatrist. In fact, the topic was not included in the first edition. McKegney[14] wrote, "It (consult-liaison [C/L]) is a provocative, but difficult to manage, promising, but largely unwanted and not very healthy offspring (of psychiatry)." Even so, I firmly believe that child psychiatrists in training must learn to be good consultants. The required skills are discussed within the context of a large pediatric hospital and its ambulatory services where I have worked for nearly 30 years. Such skills, once learned, should be easily modified for use in nonmedical settings as well.

I agree with McKegney that consultation can be provocative and difficult, but I do not agree that it is largely unwanted and unhealthy. In Prugh's[17] excellent historical overview, the relationship of child psychiatry and pediatrics is traced from Kanner in 1930 through 1978. Over the years there have been many misunderstandings and differences, but today it is clear that both pediatrics and child psychiatry seek to understand and support the child's health, growth and development. Although pediatrics has been a recognized medical discipline for over a century, child psychiatry did not emerge from the mental hospital and begin to integrate with other medical disciplines in American medical schools until about 1930. Many leading academic pediatricians and child psychiatrists have taught and tried to demonstrate the need for and usefulness of psychiatric insights in pediatric practice. This concept is no longer hotly debated or openly opposed, as it was even 20 years ago. Although psychiatric insights are at least partially accepted by pediatricians, the concepts are still not fully understood or incorporated easily into daily practice. The psychosomatic approach has influenced the field but has not fully permeated and altered practice methods. There is still a lack of widespread application of preventive measures designed to minimize the deleterious emotional reactions of children and families to surgery, illness and hospitalization. This may be particularly true for some small pediatric units in general hospitals.

In spite of increased specialization and subspecialization, many leaders in both pediatric and psychiatric education strive to teach total or comprehensive care and espouse the biopsychosocial model for the practice of medicine as an ideal. Although some training directors may give only lip service to these concepts, many are truly sincere and dedicated to making them a reality. The American Academy of Pediatrics[3] has demonstrated that young pediatricians today have considerable sophistication in psychosocial concepts and that they differ strikingly from their colleagues who completed training prior to 1960.

Hospitals and other health care delivery systems are under thoughtful pressure to change for both humanistic and economic reasons. Total care for families of children suffering chronic life-threatening and non–life-threatening illnesses has become a reality in tertiary care centers. Physicians, nurses and hospital administrators have begun paying great attention to the psychologic milieu and the physical ambiance of the hospital. The staffs are becoming family-oriented. As late as 1956 our own pediatric hospital permitted parental visitation for 2 hours only on Tuesdays and Sundays. Today, parents are present and participate in their child's treatment at all times. The

Ronald McDonald House for housing child patients' families on the medical center campus is graphic evidence that pediatrics, with the help of public and corporate philanthropy, truly acknowledges the importance of psychosocial and family influences in the treatment of sick children. In the 1950s, house officers hotly debated the issue of parental presence at the bedside. Now, discussions focus on the ways parents can be taught to help their child recover. Some parents may cause problems for the staff, but their mere presence is seldom questioned. Great advances in physiologic treatments have permitted and encouraged many pediatricians besides the few pioneers noted by Prugh to attend to psychosocial issues and child development. Psychosomatic theories have expanded to include somatopsychic concepts, and the old "organic versus functional" dilemmas have become outmoded. Pediatric training and practice have expanded from acute care to continuity of care of the chronically ill and primary prevention. Such "enlightened and modern" practices are not evident in every American community, but it is predicted they will be by the turn of the century.

Can child psychiatrists take any credit for these dramatic changes? Objective elucidation of that issue is impossible. Certainly, without vigorous, sustained effort from many enlightened, leading pediatricians no changes would have occurred. However, in a 1985 survey of practicing pediatricians, Fritz[9] found that the degree of sophistication on biopsychosocial issues and willingness to use child psychiatry consultation correlated highly with whether or not the pediatrician had had experience with child psychiatrists during residency. There is still some confusion about the roles of the behavioral pediatrician, the child psychologist and the child psychiatrist. The pediatricians also did not rate areas of expertise in the same way child psychiatrists see themselves. Yet, in Fritz's study, the difference in attitudes between those who had had psychiatric consultation available to them during training and those who had not had this experience is striking. At this time, "turf battles" between psychiatry and pediatrics seem to be looming much larger than the older battles over the usefulness of psychiatric concepts in pediatric practice.

The necessity for training in consultation is further supported by the fact that the Psychiatry Residency Review Committee has made training experience in consultation an essential requirement for both adult and child psychiatry training programs. The certifying examinations by the American Board now cover consultation in some depth. Unfortunately, many training programs have no relationships with pediatrics. Those that do, report that less than 11% of the child psychiatry fellows' time is spent in consultation activities.[8] After the promulgation of the newest "Essentials of Training" in 1986, deficiencies in training in pediatric consultation can and will adversely affect a training program's accreditation.

CONSULTATION/LIAISON

Psychiatrists seem unable to use the word *consultation* without adding word *liaison,* with a slash in between (consultation/liaison). Webster[24] defines *consultation* as talking things over in order to decide something or asking for or giving advice. This definition is consonant with consultation as it has always been practiced by physicians. The same dictionary defines *liaison* as "a linking up of parts of a whole in order to bring about proper coordination of activities." Using this definition literally would make it seem that a liaison person must inevitably come into conflict with conscientious attending physicians whose time-honored responsibility has been to link up the case findings in order to bring about proper coordination of treatment. The literature seems to be lacking a consensual definition of liaison specifically relevant to child psychiatry. National Institute for Mental Health (NIMH) has long insisted that training grants for pediatric-psychiatry programs must have a balance of liaison and consultation activities. Yet these terms are not clearly defined in the grant instructions. We might assume liaison work is similar to the consultation-consulter model described by Caplan[7] and Adams.[1] The "consulter" can be a system such as the hospital environment, the practice of medicine, physicians themselves or society at large. Adams warns us that unless we prove ourselves effective with the consultant-patient model we will never be permitted to consult with the system. Tarnow[23] defines liaison as working to modify hospital life. He recommends a systems approach. However, it is doubtful that the majority of child psychiatrists would agree that Tarnow's reforms will *a priori* promote mental health. His aim is to create "a more healthy functioning hospital system." This statement is incongruent with the limited education and training in hospital administration of the average child psychiatrist. Strain and

Grossman[22] state that the liaison psychiatrist must have knowledge of the psychologic aspects of medical illness and build alliances that will enable him to effectively transmit this knowledge to the patient's caretakers.

I prefer to follow Strain and Grossman's tenet that we must be helpful to both the patient and his caretakers. A systems approach risks having the appearance of a "reform movement." Hospitalwide changes could help some patients, make no difference to the majority and even be harmful to others. For example, a parent live-in ward has been demonstrated to reduce nursing costs, shorten the hospital stay and lessen both child and parent anxiety. It also eliminates hotel costs for parents who live too far away to commute daily. However, it is not feasible for children who require critical or intensive care. For older children and adolescents it appears to intensify undesirable child-parent dependency and at times even to increase parent-child hostility and friction. Although progress in the working relations of child psychiatry and pediatrics has been slow, they are definitely improving today and are quite tolerable in many centers. I will further describe the two models of consultation, with special attention to ways that child psychiatrist consultants can avoid excessive fatigue, role confusion and "burnout."

TWO MODELS OF CONSULTATION

Although the skills needed for the consultant-patient model and the consultant-consulter model overlap, they will be reviewed separately for clarification. The practitioner must be comfortable and proficient with both models and capable of unobtrusively shifting from one to the other or using both at the same time, depending upon the needs of the situation at hand. You must be aware of your role at all times. Give yourself time to know the hospital patient unit structure and the pediatricians individually and as a group. By personal or telephone contact find out who *really* initiated a consultation request and specifically what is wanted. Although the attending physician usually signs such requests, he/she may have been pressured to do so by a member of her/his own team. A hidden agenda may be disagreements among team members regarding diagnosis or treatment. There is no need to fear or avoid such intrastaff conflicts. Our training in psychiatric inpatient work should have made us knowledgeable as well as humble about such problems. The important point is to go into these situations with your eyes open.

The needs of the consulter and the aims of the consultant must be clarified and brought into some harmony. If the consulter hopes for some assistance with a very troublesome family, but the consultant recommends some alterations in the hospital milieu, a serious breakdown in the process may occur. I knew one academic pediatrician who had worked and taught in "his" hospital for nearly 40 years. He demanded that children and families accept the hospital as it was and vigorously opposed any changes in the milieu or in nursing procedures. The psychiatrist consultants could stay and try to work with or around this man, or they could leave. Some left. However, other consultants found that they could work with faculty pediatricians, especially during periods when the chairman was away from the wards doing his research. When changes in the milieu were imperative, patients were sometimes transferred to the children's psychiatric hospital, where psychiatrists were in charge of the milieu and the pediatricians were the consultants. Interestingly enough, this rather crotchety academic pediatrician seldom objected to such transfers. This anecdote illustrates that when the consultant-consulter model is unworkable other recommendations must be made for the sake of the patient. Such sophisticated maneuvers also require cooperation from parents and from other child psychiatrists. Of course, if the child's condition permits, it is always better to transfer him or her to outpatient psychiatric treatment, preferably in one's own clinic.

All consultants have anecdotes wherein it took considerable time to synchronize the consulter's wishes with the psychiatrist's recommendations. One house officer wrote "patient is referred for psychometrics." Direct discussion revealed that he meant "projective testing" but that he was not clear what projective testing would do for him or the child. The patient's behavior was very confusing and frustrating to him. He accepted that additional personal and family history and a mental status examination with or without a Rorschach test could probably clarify the nature of the child's mental condition and give some ideas of what would be helpful in management.

In this example we are using the consultant-patient model. The consultant collects the additional history and determines the mental status for the consulter. Then he summarizes and gives recommendations. However, if you choose to teach the consulter how to do these things with your guidance you are using the consultant-consulter model. Which model is appropriate? Experience shows that if the consulter is an overburdened, apprehensive first-year resident or a practitioner who has never learned these procedures, it is best to follow the consultant-patient model. Some seasoned residents and practitioners want us to help them refine their own skills in this area and actually prefer the consultant-consulter approach. However, you should never frustrate yourself by trying to teach persons who are not ready or willing to learn. One must always ask the consulter whether he wishes you to take charge of the workup and management or just to give advice.

In addition to knowing both consultation models and being flexible, consultants must be available, practical and understandable. Coupled with your written response in the patient's chart you must give the consulter full confidential feedback. A follow-up contact with the consulter in 48 to 96 hours is very important to learn whether the recommendation is feasible and whether anything else is needed.[16] This is true whether you are advising on a patient or the system.

Having "trouble identifying the psychiatrist's unique social usefulness" can be a serious handicap for a consultant. If you suffer those feelings, do something about them. Literally everyone from the dock worker to the president of the United States knows *the* answer to the emotionally and behaviorally disordered child. You are unique in that you know that there is no *one* answer and you have the humility to say you do not know and the willingness to try to find answers. In 1952, G.A.P.[11] reviewed five areas in which relevant knowledge from child psychiatry can be useful in clinical pediatric practice. These are knowledge of (1) personality development; (2) interview techniques; (3) child-parent-physician relationships; (4) psychologic and social reactions of children and families to physical illness, hospitalization, surgery or convalescence; and (5) psychopathology and symptom formation. Many other professional disciplines have some or even all of that knowledge. However, you are practicing the only medical discipline for which knowledge in those five areas is fundamental to your basic training in a clinical setting. In the years since the G.A.P.'s 1952 report, knowledge in each of these five areas has expanded significantly. Today's child psychiatrists also have much more knowledge about prognosis and many more forms of treatment than their counterparts in 1952 had. The child psychiatrist consultant needs to learn how to apply and impart that knowledge effectively.

THE CONSULTANT-PATIENT–CENTERED CONSULTATIONS

A practice employing consultant-patient–centered consultants can be exhausting and overwhelming from the large number of referrals that may occur in a week. There may be little time for teaching. Our supervisors and some funding agencies seem to look more favorably upon a systems approach, perhaps because it is more difficult, more abstract and more nearly utopian in its potential benefit for humankind. Sometimes it may seem that our pediatric colleagues are just "dumping" troublesome or unwanted cases upon us and have no interest in learning psychiatric principles to apply to the next case. Another problem is that time will not permit you to become the personal psychotherapist for all of the children for whom you recommend such treatment. Sometimes your careful and thoughtful advice may be rejected or ignored. Consultation requests often come at inconvenient times, and it may seem that the consulters do not appreciate the pressures on your time. Fee collections for consultations are often poor. Such are some of the problems with using the consultant-patient model.

In spite of all the negative agents that may frustrate and lessen the professional gratification of the consultant, patient consultation work can be quite enjoyable. It is a good practice builder for the young clinician. If you take care to be sure the parents know who you are, find out how they plan to pay, have your office bill promptly within 48 hours and send follow-up bills, delinquent accounts are only slightly higher than in other aspects of practice. Obtaining significant patient improvement from short-term psychotherapy, clarification of the issues, or alterations in medication often occurs and is pleasurable for the family, the pediatrician and the psychiatrist. Certainly, practicing pediatricians and their patients need and deserve the best we have to offer. We must offer more than just triage or instruction.

In former times, the so-called case dumpers offended and annoyed me. Now I truly believe that such persons are educationally and temperamentally unsuited for helping with psychosocial problems and that it is in the best interest of the child that he be referred promptly to a psychiatrist. Contrary to popular belief, it is my experience that in established consultation services referrals at inconvenient times or only after all physical studies are completed occur less and less frequently. If I could not solve those two problems, i.e., inconvenient and "end-of-the-line" referrals, in 30 years, I would deserve to suffer burnout. The patients in many of the pediatric subspecialty clinics have a high incidence of secondary or concomitant emotional problems. Their staffs know this, and families are informed of the likelihood of a psychiatric consultation at the time of admission. Psychiatric consultation requests usually are sent long before the physical findings are complete. A 1985 survey by Fritz[10] shows the volume of requests is rather even throughout the week, with the smallest number occurring on Friday afternoons and seldom after 4:30 p.m. If the psychiatrist assigned a consultation does not have time to see the patient the same day the request arrives, he/she must telephone the consulter to inquire whether an emergency exists. The consultant must be able to reassure the consulter that the patient will be seen as soon as possible, ask one of his colleagues to take the case, or work late. If the consulter wants the patient seen immediately because discharge is imminent, I arrange to conduct the consultation in the outpatient clinic within a week after discharge. I have no data on how frequently my advice is rejected or ignored. The only way one can be certain that one's recommendations are followed is to become the primary case manager oneself. This is often not necessary, advisable or feasible. Rejection does occur, and one must learn that a consultation service is not the place "to wear one's feelings on one's sleeve." When I recommend continued therapy with someone else, a placement or a special education program, my office or I arranges those referrals as part of the consultation with the knowledge and consent of the parents and the consulter. Additional fees are charged for these services. With this approach, I at least know that my advice is not ignored and also learn when it is rejected. My practice has a knowledge of community resources that is naturally broader than that of the average pediatric resident. With their busy ward schedules and relative lack of secretarial assistance for letter writing and telephoning they welcome our help. I also try to teach them to enlist collaboration from the hospital social work department or the mental health nurse specialists in setting up after-care plans.

Time—or lack of it—is an ominous enemy of the consultant. Some chiefs of child psychiatry assign one psychiatrist, often the newest staff member, to "do the consultations," an unrealistic practice unless the pediatric service is an extremely small one. The consultant also has the obligation to protect her/his physical and mental well-being. You must have time to study, to be the primary therapist for some patients, to teach and to perform other activities essential for your own professional development. The pressures and the schedule disruptions of an active consultant service mandate that the consultant have assistance from colleagues in psychiatry as well as other disciplines. Doing it all oneself on a full-time basis is a certain path to burnout.

CONSULTANT-CONSULTER–CENTERED CONSULTATIONS

Direct patient consultation often requires changing the hospital milieu (system) to support treatment or to a primary treatment modality. I never recommend that the consulter change the hospital. Rather, I offer to meet with him/her, the nurses and other staff to try to bring about changes in the milieu and/or devise a ward care plan. Often staff are willing to try to change for specific goals with particular patients, and dramatic results do come about. However, if the patient does not respond in a reasonable length of time or if the environment is too resistive, psychiatric hospitalization of the child may be necessary. Criticizing or scapegoating the staff is usually counterproductive. After all, even in very sophisticated psychiatric hospitals, milieu therapy can be most difficult to institute and maintain. The milieu therapy program for any child or group of children requires constant monitoring by the physician with knowledge of the treatment principles, considerable team leadership ability and adequate final authority. In the nonpsychiatric hospital the consultant's authority or "clout" rests entirely within his/her relationship with the attending pediatricians.

The reader is no doubt aware from statements made earlier in this chapter that I dislike the word *liaison* and do not always approve of the way the liaison role is practiced by colleagues. On the other hand, primary prevention is a highly desirable goal. Yet, primary prevention on a mass basis producing a discernible effect seems like something that will occur only in the Utopia of the millennium. It is very difficult to obtain funding for both liaison and primary prevention, mostly because positive results, if they do occur, do so in years rather than days or weeks. They are also products of concepts that our consumers (other physicians) and society at large have not really wanted. The concepts have come to sound like platitudes. This is not surprising if you consider that even with the child labor laws and other reform movements of this century, the incidence of infanticide and child abuse may be only somewhat lower than it was in the Middle Ages. Prior to the mid-1920s, adoption laws were concerned only with the transfer of property and titles, and no concerns about the humanistic needs of children or prospective parents were attended. In the 19th century, long before child psychiatry was known as a medical specialty, many persons tried to improve the "system" or society in which children were raised. One of the most notable was Charles Dickens. These illustrations are a way of saying the psychiatric consultant can, perhaps should, use the consulter-consultant model to try to change the system, whether it is pediatric practices or hospital environments, but with modest goals. Some successes and many failures will occur, and the utmost in patience and perseverance is needed.

An in-depth review of the literature and my own experience fail to disclose a "sure-fire" way of making an impact on the system. Therefore, I will only give an account of the development of our pediatric-child psychiatry consultation program with the hope that the reader can pick out a few principles that suit his/her own temperament and clinical setting.

In 1953, I became a part-time member of the child psychiatry faculty of the Indiana University School of Medicine and a staff member of Indiana University Hospitals, which include the James Whitcomb Riley Hospital for Children. In 1958, I joined the psychiatry faculty full-time and agreed to "coordinate" the psychiatry residents' training in child psychiatry and to try to improve the psychiatric-pediatric consultation activities. I was given an office in the child guidance clinic located in the Riley Hospital as well as an office in the Children's Residential Unit of an adjacent hospital. Visibility and availability are prime requisites for a consultant. Also, psychiatric inpatient beds for children too disturbed to be managed on an open pediatric ward may be necessary.

In 1958, the Pediatric Department had been pressuring for psychiatric services for some time, but what did they want? It quickly became evident that they did not want to be changed or reformed. They did want assistance with differential diagnosis, help in curtailing the behavior of children whose psychosocial problems impinged on the system and removal to our psychiatric hospital of those children who could not be comfortably managed on the open pediatric wards.[21] I did what they asked. Purist liaison persons might call my behavior, at worst, pandering or, at best, a serious compromise of principles. I did not think much about it at the time, because I was too busy. In retrospect, I think that I was responding to my own survival instincts. Once in 1954, I had refused to let my critically ill daughter be hospitalized at Riley because I did not like the way resident and faculty pediatricians related to the children and felt that the restriction of parental visits to Tuesday and Sunday afternoons was an abomination. Even though I was told that faculty members did not have to abide by the rules, my child was admitted to a small pediatric unit in a private general hospital, where the pediatrician of our choosing treated her and where one or the other of her parents could be in attendance at all times. I could not have endured that experience otherwise. My protest went largely unnoticed by both the pediatric and psychiatric faculty. I was only part-time on the faculty, was not sure I wanted to stay at the University and did not care to call attention to myself with a loud protest about the "system."

The 9 years between 1958 and 1967 were often difficult and tiring, but I was pleased that my fatigue was due to the large number of consultation referrals and a heavy teaching load, not to faculty in-fighting. I believed that I was helping many children who for a variety of reasons could or would not come to the psychiatric clinic. Our psychiatry residents were getting a good pediatric experience. Some of the pediatric residents and faculty were knowledgeable and interested in the biopsychosocial model for pediatric practice. We enjoyed practicing and teaching, and we learned from each other. In the early 1960s, the hospital milieu did change as children were permitted out of their beds and away from their wards and parental visitation was gradually liberalized. I had the privilege of working on a few hospital committees and planning groups. I was pleased with the changes that have occurred but have no memory of ever being the instigator of change. Perhaps I could only use the consultant-consulter model or be a liaison person when I was not conscious that I was doing it. In the late 1960s, the dean appointed me chairman of a multidisciplinary faculty advisory committee for the planning of a new construction of Riley Hospital. He said that I was needed because he knew I could "pour oil on troubled waters" and I had a reputation for helping differing factions reach compromise. He emphasized that I was to serve as a faculty member and not as a psychiatrist consultant for the Advisory Committee. I have also been welcomed as a consultant for groups of highly stressed medical teams such as those described by Maloney.[13] John Reinhart, Mike Jellinek, other child psychiatrists and I have worked "by invitation" with the American Academy of Pediatrics Committee on the psychosocial aspects of child and family health. Over the years I have met a number of child psychiatry colleagues who seem to be working comfortably in pediatric settings, but these persons do not tend to make themselves visible in the literature.

Perhaps I did not initiate changes because I did not have to. In 1967, Dr. Morris Green was appointed chairman of pediatrics. We had worked together in the clinics and on the wards for several years. His prior work and study experiences with such vanguards of the psychosocial model and of comprehensive care as Milton Seen, Al Solnit, Julius Richmond and others were always in evidence. Morris Green came as a breath of fresh air. His predecessor had seemed to tolerate child psychiatry out of necessity, not out of any understanding or respect for our clinical skills. The stories I have heard about serious conflicts between child psychiatrists and pediatric chairmen at some centers are alien to me and, at times, shocking. Basically, we are all pledged to the best care for children. Differences over what is "the best" should not cause deep schisms, but they do. I would never have psychologically burned out, but neither would I have stayed at Indiana University if I had suffered some of the abuses my colleagues recount. Perhaps these are just "war stories" that are commonly recounted over drinks by the "old soldier buddies" at the annual "Legion" (psychiatric) convention.

During the 18 years of Morris Green's chairmanship, the psychologic milieu and the physical ambiance of the hospital have changed drastically. The younger faculty accept psychosocial precepts and comprehensive care to the best of their individual abilities. The "old guard" has left. In 1954, I could not let my own seriously ill child be treated in Riley Hospital. Today, should the need arise, I would not want one of my grandchildren treated anywhere else. I feel a part of the establishment, a new establishment, and I would probably join the resistance against any young insurgents who might want to change us now. After all, a hospital or a medical specialty can probably survive a revolution only once every other generation.

I have not personally directed the Riley pediatric-child psychiatry consultation service since 1981, but I still work there and take consultation requests 1 day per week. The service is alive and reasonably healthy. Of course, improvements and changes are needed. Ideally, these can be made in due time without the pediatricians', the child psychiatrists' or their child patients' suffering any serious developmental delays or regressions.

SUMMARY

In consultation practice the psychiatrist may use the consultant-patient model or the consultant-consulter model. At times he or she may need to use both models in a given situation. For a variety of very pragmatic reasons, the child psychiatrists must be trained in the skillful use of both models. A brief review of the relationship between pediatrics and child psychiatry over the past 55 years is offered and significant improvements with many lingering problems are noted.

I reject the term *liaison psychiatry* partly because I cannot find a clear definition of it and partly because I believe that it has too often been detrimental and counterproductive to true collaboration of pediatricians and psychiatrists. Being human, pediatricians seem to accept and request help on patients and issues that pose problems for them but react negatively to consultants who try to tell them how to practice pediatrics better.

The unique social usefulness of child psychiatry is described in terms of its knowledge base. The need for child psychiatrists to learn to apply and impart that knowledge effectively for others is underscored. Lack of time is our constant enemy and its judicious use is vital. The process of patient-centered consultation is described in some detail. As an overview of my personal use of the consultant-consulter model indicates, I have enjoyed collaboration with many pediatricians but have shunned or side-stepped activities intended to change the many social systems that impinge upon children. It is readily acknowledged that social changes have always been and will always be critically needed for children. I have merely chosen to leave that task for the most courageous and dedicated among us. Some suggestions for careful allocation of time and special attention to one's own professional growth and development along with focusing on realistic goals are offered to help the psychiatrist consultant avoid early burnout and a deep sense of failure as a consultant. The turf battles we see on the horizon now are apparently not so much a conflict over the usefulness of psychiatric principles as a concern with personal egos and economic issues. Perhaps that's the price psychiatry must pay for the acceptance of psychosocial tenets and their use in medical practice.

I know that I have had many dark and discouraging moments in my work as a consultant. It is tempting to try to cite them as teaching vignettes, but the readers' frustrations will be different. You, the new generation of child psychiatrists, seem brighter and are certainly more thoroughly trained than we were. You will find your way.

REFERENCES

1. Adams, P.L.: Techniques for pediatric consultation, in Schwab, J.J. (Ed.). *Handbook of Psychiatric Consultation.* New York, Appleton Century Crofts, 1968, pp. 107–138.
2. Ahsanuddin, K.M. and Adams, J.E.: Setting up a pediatric consultation liaison service. Psychiatr. Clin. North American, *5*:259–270, 1982.
3. American Academy of Pediatrics: Survey of Practicing Pediatricians, personal communication, 1982.
4. Anders, T.F.: Child psychiatry and pediatrics: The state of the relationship. Pediatrics, *60*:616, 1977.
5. Berlin, I.N.: Mental health consultation to child-serving agencies as therapeutic intervention, in *Basic Handbook of Child Psychiatry.* Vol. 3. Noshpitz, J.D. (Ed.). New York, Basic Books, 1979.
6. Caplan, G.: Recent trends in preventive child psychiatry, Chapter 7 in *Emotional Problems of Early Childhood,* Caplan, G. (Ed.). New York, Basic Book, Inc., 1955.
7. Caplan, G.: *Principles of Preventive Psychiatry.* New York, Basic Books, Inc., 1964.
8. Fritz, G.K. and Bergman, A.S.: Consultation-liaison training for child psychiatrists: Results of a survey. Gen. Hosp. Psychiatry, *6*:25–29, 1984.
9. Fritz, G.K. and Bergman, A.S.: Child psychiatrists seen through pediatri-

cians' eyes: Results of a national survey. J. Am. Acad. Child Psychiatry, *24*:81–87, 1985.

10. Fritz, J.K.: Timing of requests for child psychiatry consultation: Perception and reality, personal communication, 1985.

11. Group for the Advancement of Psychiatry: *The Contribution of Child Psychiatry to Pediatric Training and Practice.* New York, G.A.P., Report No. 21, 1952.

12. Lewis, M.: Child psychiatric consultation in pediatrics. Pediatr., *62*:359–364, 1978.

13. Maloney, M.J. and Auge, C.: Group consultation with highly stressed medical personnel to avoid burnout. Acad. Child Psychiatry, *121*:481–485, 1982.

14. McKegney, P.F.: Consultation-liaison teaching of psychosomatic medicine: Opportunities and obstacles. J. Nerv. Ment. Dis., *154*:198–205, 1972.

15. Perry, S. and Viederman, M.: Adaptation of residents to consultation liaison psychiatry, II. Gen. Hosp. Psychiatry, *3*:149–156, 1981.

16. Popkin, M., Mackenzie, T., and Callies, A.: Improving the effectiveness of psychiatric consultation. Psychosomatics, *22*:559–563, 1981.

17. Prugh, D.G. and Eckhardt, L.O.: Child psychiatry and pediatrics, in *Basic Handbook of Child Psychiatry.* Noshpitz, J.D. (Ed.). New York, Basic Books, 1979, pp. 563–576.

18. Roeske, N.C.A.: Education of the Paraprofessional in *Basic Handbook of Child Psychiatry,* Noshpitz, J.D. (Ed.). New York, Basic Books, Vol. IV. 1979, pp. 511–518.

19. Rothenberg, M.B.: Child psychiatry-pediatrics liaison: A history and commentary. J. Am. Acad. Child Psychiatry, *7*:492–509, 1968.

20. Rothenberg, M.B.: Child psychiatry-pediatrics consultation liaison services in the hospital setting. Gen. Hosp. Psychiatry, *1*:281–286, 1979.

21. Sack, W.H. and Blicker, D.L.: Who gets referred? Child psychiatric consultation in a pediatric hospital. Int. J. Psychiatry in Medicine, *9*:329–337, 1979.

22. Strain, J.J. and Grossman, S.: *Psychological Care of the Medically Ill.* New York, Appleton-Century-Crofts, 1975, pp. 3–11.

23. Tarnow, J.D. and Gutstein, S.E.: Systemic consultation in a general hospital. Intl. J. Psychiatry in Med., *12*:161–186, 1982.

24. *Webster's New World Dictionary,* 2d. College Ed. New York, The World Publishing Co., 1976.

25. Wise, T.N. and Berlin, R.M.: Burnout: Stress in consultation-liaison psychiatry. Psychosomatics *22*:(9), 744–751, 1981.

12

THE INTERFACE BETWEEN PEDIATRICS AND CHILD PSYCHIATRY

The previous chapter on consultation reviewed a great deal about the relationship between pediatrics and child psychiatry. However, there are several important issues in addition to the consulting and referral processes. The following discussion will review what I see as current practices and the kinds of relationships we hope might develop in the future for continually improving patient care.

Perhaps it would be appropriate to have a thesis about child psychiatry's interface with all medical specialties, not just pediatrics. Ideally, many of the concepts reviewed herein can readily be extrapolated for use by other specialties, particularly family practice. Many leaders in pediatric education have adopted the position that training in pediatrics shall include the development of considerable expertise in the diagnosis and management of mental, emotional and behavioral disorders in children and adolescents.[2] To the best of our knowledge, the other specialties have not been so specific regarding training in child mental health.

LACK OF EFFECTIVE WORKING RELATIONSHIPS

Logic might indicate that our mutual interest in the well-being of children would have brought pediatrics and child psychiatry into a very close, positive liaison. Even though this has not occurred with many older members of the two specialties, younger physicians and the next generation show more promise of being able to collaborate. In medical centers where the two specialties do work together, fewer and fewer students and house officers seem confused about psychosocial issues, and they no longer question whether or not emotional and behavior problems are the responsibility of the medically trained clinician. In the private practice sector, parents are consulting their child's pediatrician about school problems and a wide range of social, emotional and developmental issues. A telephone survey of 1,201 mothers by the Task Force on Pediatric Education[2] found that 20 per cent of the total surveyed had had some biosocial or developmental problems (behavioral, learning and emotional problems included) with their child. They reported turning most often to their child's pediatrician for help. The vast majority felt that the consultation had been helpful, and they expressed a willingness to pay for the extra amount of physician's time required.

Pediatricians are seeing increasing numbers of adolescents, an age group well known for its high emotionality and in which the interaction of psyche and soma is intense and not easily disconnected. Tremendous technical advances in surgery and medicine have reduced infant and child mortality and made it possible for chronically ill or handicapped children not only to live, but to participate in the mainstream of society. Many of these children present a host of difficult psychologic and developmental enigmas to their primary care physician. The 1977 personnel survey by the American Academy of Pediatrics[3] documented significant increase in the amount of time pediatricians are spending in counseling for school problems. Most practitioners seem to welcome these new challenges. Some do not.

The Task Force[3] surveyed by letter all members of the American Academy of Pediatrics who had graduated from medical school in 1961 or thereafter. More than 90% of this group practice general pediatrics. Nearly 16% had a special interest in behavioral and psychosocial problems. Only neonatal/perinatal medicine held a higher special interest rate (20.9%). Over one-half of the total respondents felt that their residency training in psychosocial and behavioral problems was "insufficient." It is of interest that this negative rating of insufficient training in biosocial matters dropped to less than 33% of those completing residency by 1975–77. This illustrates a rather radical change in pediatric training. Even so, 72.6% stated they do provide such services as counseling or management of learning disorders and of other psychosocial problems. My own observation is that although many more pediatricians feel a responsibility to attend to their patients' emotional/behavioral problems, noncompliance with treatment, parental psychopathology and family disequilibrium remain as serious enigmas.

Child psychiatry as a subspecialty of general psychiatry only received official recognition in the late 1950s. As such, it is one of the newest and numerically smallest specialties in medicine. Just prior to the establishment of a Subcommittee on Child Psychiatry within the American Board of Psychiatry and Neurology, there were strong pro and con arguments about child psychiatry's more appropriately being a subspecialty of pediatrics. Prior to World War II, pediatric training was largely restricted to physiologic or organic disease problems, whereas psychiatry concentrated its efforts on more purely psychologic or functional problems. Pediatricians have traditionally worked within the medical setting and the medical community; whereas child psychiatrists have been located more often in social or public health types of settings. In the 1930s a few child psychiatrists were on medical school faculties, but not until the 1960s did most medical schools make a concerted effort to bring child psychiatry into the curriculum. Like the prodigal son, child psychiatry left home (the medical clinic and hospital). Unlike the prodigal son, the child psychiatrist found that when he tried to return home there was no accepting, loving, protecting father there and the siblings were highly ambivalent about letting him in.

The two requisites for effective cooperation are geographic proximity and continuing dialogue. The distance between child psychiatry and pediatrics is not the result of any deliberate act by anyone. Rather, it is a happenstance of the times. As Rothenberg pointed out in 1968,[4] there could never be a relationship until the two professions could meet and talk with each other on curriculum committees and in case conferences. Such interchanges do occur at some centers. Unfortunately, many medical schools still have no full-time child psychiatrist faculty and no visible child psychiatric services. Current pressure from the residency review committee of both pediatrics and psychiatry through the Liaison Council for Graduate Medical Education may change this deficiency.

BEHAVIORAL PEDIATRICS

Pediatricians' overall dissatisfaction with child psychiatric services, both quantitatively and qualitatively, has probably contributed to interest in the new subspecialty of "behavioral pediatrics." Some pediatricians remaining true to their early training are singularly "organically minded." They may refuse to acknowledge the importance of psychosocial phenomena to the development of their patients. However, more likely, they believe that such problems are not the responsibility of pediatrics and require immediate referral to a child psychiatrist or some other mental health professional. There are some pediatricians who feel that they should personally handle every problem of every patient. A more middle-of-the-road position is that pediatricians should be able to do many things, including managing most of the biologic, psychologic and social problems that affect their patients, but that the pediatrician cannot and should not be expected to do everything. The pediatrician should liberally use all types of medical consultations and professionals from other disciplines outside medicine to assure total care and effective management for the problems of the developing child. In fact, achieving skill in obtaining the assistance of nonmedical specialists in psychology, social work, education, law and many other professions concerned with the care of children probably has to be included in the training of the pediatrician of the future.[5]

Most physicians want to do something practical for the troubled children in their own daily practice. The primary physician is expected by the public and by his colleagues to be able to diagnose a delay in development, a functional disorder of any organ system, mood and behavior disorders, learning disorders and a host of other psychologic and psychosomatic phenomena. He is expected either to cure or alleviate these conditions or to make an intelligent referral to some professional who can. The numbers of children requiring help with behavioral, emotional and learning problems and those with combined chronic mental and physical problems seem to be steadily increasing for most practitioners. Those who advocate the establishment of a new subspecialty of behavioral pediatrics are sincere in their belief that such a trained group is crucially needed today. They offer in evidence the painfully slow development of child psychiatry as a subspecialty and this latter group's continued inability to provide the quantity of service needed. However, there are others who fear that another subspecialty will not only fail to relieve the trained staff shortage but truly compound professional schisms and the fractionated health care delivery of the past. This latter group, to which the author subscribes, believes that a better answer lies in teaching all physicians, especially those in primary care, the principles of biopsychosocial medical practice and the developmental approach to the care of children. Behavioral pediatricians are still too few in number to present an immediate economic threat to child psychiatrists. They are, or will be, yet another professional group that purports to have psychiatric skills, thereby disturbing child psychiatry's concept of its unique social usefulness. There is some evidence[1] that pediatric house officers want to learn biopsychosocial principles but that they do not wish to limit their practices to behavior problems.

The idea of instilling the principles of biopsychosocial developmental medicine into the minds of every medical student may seem even more quixotic than the idea of creating yet another medical subspecialty. However, should the medical establishment reach a consensus on this matter, it is quite possible that the interactions of individuals within a family in a given social matrix can be discovered and learned over time as easily as the relationships among various physiologic systems within the human body.

EFFECTIVE WORKING RELATIONSHIPS

Physicians' interests, attitudes, skills and training backgrounds, plus the kinds of problems presented by patients, are all much too variable to permit any rigid categorization of which patient should see whom and which physician should be permitted to do what. The significant overlapping of talents and skills among physicians with different training backgrounds further renders such categorization impossible. Developing children, especially those with chronic illnesses, need expert physiologic and psychologic care. Each new crisis or problem must be carefully studied to decide whether the pediatrician or the psychiatrist alone should assume full responsibility or whether they must manage the situation together. The prognosis of the child's condition can serve as one guideline for such decisions. The many factors contributing to prognosis and a method of prognosticating are offered next. The responsibility for obtaining the data upon which prognosis is based rests with the pediatrician who wishes to offer comprehensive care. It is almost always the pediatrician or the primary care physician who is consulted first. Thus, it is usually impossible for the child psychiatrist to participate in the data-gathering process unless requested to do so by the pediatrician. If there is a close working relationship between the pediatrician and child psychiatrist, informal conferences are, of course, possible and often helpful.

PROGNOSTICATING: A PRELIMINARY TO TREATMENT

Prognosticating on a case-by-case basis is essential to any treatment planning. The same data used in deciding a prognosis are also helpful in deciding whether the long-term or ongoing case management should rest primarily with the pediatrician or the child psychiatrist. Unfortunately, statistics on children with similar problems are useless in prognosticating. There are simply too many variables contributing to outcome. The 1980 *DSM-III* has been and will probably continue to be a great assistance to physicians in diagnosis. Although many of these diagnostic entities are empirically known to carry a relatively good or bad prognosis, there are often, if not usually, other factors of equal or even greater importance than the diagnostic label in predicting treatability.

In the context used here, "case-by-case prognostication" is simply deciding, Is this a child I can help on an outpatient basis in my office, with the skills and time I have at my disposal? The following variables must be considered in intelligent prognostication:

1. Severity of the problem(s)
2. Chronicity of the problem(s)
3. The child's premorbid adjustment
4. The ability of the child to engage meaningfully with the physician and/or to work on the problem(s)
5. The ability of both parents to participate actively in the treatment
6. The number of other problems in the family and overall stability of the family
7. The physician's attitudes toward
   A. This child
   B. The type of problem this child has
   C. The family
   D. His own (the physician's) abilities

The aim of reviewing each of the preceding prognostic variables is to give some objective criteria that the pediatrician can use in deciding, Should I, personally, try to help this youngster or should I refer the case, and, if so, to whom, where?

CONDITIONS ESSENTIAL FOR PROGNOSTICATION

Although any of the preceding seven parameters of prognostication may be a decisive factor in determining outcome, none can stand alone in all cases. To be successful, the pediatrician should not jump to conclusions about the treatability of a condition without a careful examination to obtain a minimal data base on these items. The procedure requires that the pediatrician have the interest, the time and the interviewing skills necessary for at least minimal psychiatric diagnostic screening.

Although it has not been confirmed by a large number of pediatricians, it is estimated that a minimal screening takes 1 to 2 hours of a pediatrician's time in most instances. This amount of time, of course, does not have to be in a day or in one appointment but probably is better done in shorter visits, scattered over several days or weeks, unless there is some undue urgency or emergency.

In the preceding chapters, I have reviewed in detail what constitutes a complete psychiatric examination of a child, and the outline for the total case study is presented in Chapter 9. It is acknowledged that the complete psychiatric examination of a significant number of children is too cumbersome and impractical for the busy schedule of the average primary care physician. Minimal screening differs from a complete psychiatric evaluation, not only in that it takes much less time, but in that its aim is only to obtain enough information to assess severity and probable treatability. A more extensive psychiatric examination is, of course, needed if one intends to assume full responsibility for eliciting all probable causes and for long-range treatment.

In addition to the usual health history and physical examination, the elements for a minimal screening with estimated time required are as follows.

1. Review of the presenting emotional problem or social problems and antecedents with the child and both parents: 10 to 12 minutes
2. Review of the child's birth and social-emotional ad-

justment up to the time of present symptoms: 5 to 10
minutes

3. Review of family relations and stability
   A. Interview with mother: 15 minutes
   B. Interview with father: 15 minutes
4. Partial mental status of the child—a series of two to
   four 15- to 20-minute interviews (30 to 80 minutes) at
   weekly intervals to assess
   A. Conventionality or lack of it in the child's thinking
   B. Child's understanding or insight into his/her prob-
      lems
   C. Child's attitude(s) toward accepting professional
      help (ability to share thoughts and feelings with
      doctor)
   D. Child's ability to maintain usual daily activities
      while receiving treatment
5. Review of the child's school adjustment (obtained by
   a questionnaire mailed to the school; see Chapter 10):
   total 75 to 132 minutes

Lack of time is one of the principal reasons that many pediatricians do not offer treatment for psychosocial problems.
They are right. No physician should ever offer services if he/
she does not have the time to perform them properly. Yet, with
the data obtained in the outlined interviews, we can often see
that some cases can be managed more easily and effectively
than others. Minimal screening is used only to help the primary
physician decide whether he should try to work with the child
and family himself or should refer the case.

The following chart cannot be quantified in absolutes but is
offered as a guide to help primary care physicians screen children for office treatment of behavioral or emotional problems.

Prognosis Guide		
	Finding usually points toward a good outcome	Finding usually points toward a poor outcome or necessity for long arduous treatment
Severity of problem(s)	Symptoms may be somatic but are non–life-threatening	Life-threatening to self or others
	Symptoms uncomfortable to child or family but not inca-pacitating	Behavior dangerous or illegal Symptoms disrupting to usual social, school, or work func-tioning

Prognosis Guide *Continued*

	Finding usually points toward a good outcome	Finding usually points toward a poor outcome or necessity for long arduous treatment
	Symptoms in one area only; i.e., school, home, society (including friends, personal well-being)	Symptoms in all four areas
Chronicity	Symptoms less than 6 months' duration	Symptoms persisting longer than 6 months or chronically recurring over several years
	Precipitating stress(es) obvious with clear-cut onset of symptoms	Precipitating stress(es) unclear and onset vague or insidious
Child's premorbid adjustment	Has had good physical health	Many minor or major physical problems since conception
	Developmental milestones within normal range	Development delayed or erratic
	Good relationship with both parents and relatively few discipline problems	Poor relations with one or both parents—clinging, overcompliant or rebellious
	Smooth progression in preschool and primary grades, academically and socially	Erratic or chronically poor school performance
	Has friendships with peers	No friends or only social deviants
	Has friendships with adults	Intimidated by or defiant of adults
Child's ability to "engage" with physician	Talks easily about non–emotion-laden topics	Does not talk at all or rattles on about superficial matters for as long as four visits
	With encouragement and time can discuss feelings and other confidential matters	Steadfastly distrusts physician for as long as four visits
	May blame others but considers his own contribution to the problems	Projects blame without slightest consideration of own role in the problems
	Can state own views even though they may not be conventional	States only what he thinks examiner wishes to hear for as long as four visits
	Is serious but maintains a sense of humor	No sense of humor or is inappropriately glib or silly
	May be discouraged but hasn't given up hope	Persists with feelings of hopelessness
	Has the capacity to like himself and others	Has no friends and nothing good to say about himself
Parents' ability to participate in treatment	Both parents are willing to come with child for appointments, as indicated	One or both parents resent giving the time, fail appointments, or make excuses

Prognosis Guide *Continued*

	Finding usually points toward a good outcome	Finding usually points toward a poor outcome or necessity for long arduous treatment
	Parents seek advice but don't monopolize doctor	Parent(s) monopolize doctor's time or argue with most suggestions
	Parents pay bills promptly and facilitate child's transportation	Parents are vague about financial arrangements and find transporting child a burden
	Parents share responsibility	One parent has abdicated responsibility
	Parents seek/accept marital counseling, if indicated	Parents persistently use sessions to fix blame on each other
	Parents voluntarily sought help	Parents were *forced* to seek help by a social agency
	Both parents are free of serious social and mental problems	One or both parents suffer from mental illness or alcoholism
	Parents are not seriously considering divorce	One or both parents having an affair or seriously seeking divorce
	If divorced, matters of custody, visitation and support are relatively settled	If divorced, matters of custody, visitation and support are a constant battle
Stability of family	Relatively little history of mental illness or serious social problems among grandparents, aunts and uncles	Family history replete with mental and social problems
	Siblings have few problems	Siblings have so many problems you wonder why only one child was brought to you
	Vocational stability of parents	Frequent job changes
	Residential stability Family crises handled quickly and smoothly	Frequent family moves Family seems to live in a state of chronic crisis
Physician's attitude(s)	Physician likes the child or believes he will come to like him	Physician dislikes child and has trouble knowing why
	Physician likes or respects most of the family members	Physician dislikes the family or has trouble finding any redeeming features about them
	Physician is not shocked, repulsed, angered or fearful about child's symptoms	Child's symptoms create considerable inner discomfort in the physician

Prognosis Guide *Continued*

Finding usually points toward a good outcome	Finding usually points toward a poor outcome or necessity for long arduous treatment
Physician would like to try to treat this child (family)	Physician fears that he/she is not capable of helping this family

Note: Information relevant to each of the preceding items can seldom, if ever, be obtained during one office visit. Keep in mind that many children are suspicious and uncommunicative at the first visit. Therefore, judgment on the items under "Child's ability to 'engage' with the physician" should be deferred until the third or fourth visit.

The preceding chart obviously contains the extremes at each end of a treatability scale. We have not tried to quantify these items on a scale of 1 to 5, or a scale of 1 to 10, to try to get a numerical score. However, if the child and his family score in the left-hand column on every item, the symptoms will probably abate spontaneously, so it is safe to offer only reassurance. On the other hand, if they score consistently in the right-hand column, outpatient office therapy will be extremely difficult, and perhaps impossible, even by the most skilled clinician. In between the two extremes, it is likely that a majority of practicing pediatricians would find some cases that they would feel comfortable in treating in their own office before making a referral.

WHEN TO REFER

Office therapy of children's emotional and behavior problems is nearly always a calculated risk in terms of outcome. The tedium of continuously exploring for cause(s) and the slowness in bringing about changes can cause considerable pressure on the clinician. Human resistance to change and the long plateaus that so often occur in the therapy of children with emotional problems make even the most expert clinician wonder at times whether there is someone, somewhere, who could do it better and faster. Many pediatricians are rightfully reluctant to involve themselves in management of a case that might result in unbearable tedium or appear to be increasingly complex as time goes on, without some assurance that a referral to a child psychiatrist can be made in the future. Certainly, such a referral should be considered before the pediatrician and the family decide that they have failed completely, and it should be made if—

1. the symptoms become worse or remain unchanged for more than 90 days;
2. behavior becomes seriously disruptive to ordinary office routines;
3. the situation becomes increasingly complex, with too many family problems requiring too much time and attention;
4. suicidal tendencies, physical changes, or custody, placement and other sociologic problems become evident; and/or
5. unremitting discomfort of the physician or the family develops.

How effective the outlined procedures would be for selecting children to be treated in the general pediatrician's office depends, to a large extent, upon the pediatrician's interest and his proficiency in biopsychosocial medical practice, plus his respect for and confidence in his child psychiatric colleagues. The child psychiatrist must be visible and available to his pediatric colleagues and, of course, must agree that minimal screening and at least tentative prognostication truly belong within the province of the general pediatrician. It is really not a matter of under whose jurisdiction the child's illness falls. It is more correctly a problem of finding how and by whom the child can most expeditiously and effectively be helped.

The principles upon which the preceding theses are based certainly are not new in the history of medicine. The primary care physician does not refer simple, nutritional anemias to the hematology or oncology subspecialist. However, he certainly does refer the malignant blood dyscrasias. In between these two simple examples, there are many patients with hematologic abnormalities that the physician might feel quite competent to treat himself, or to whom he would want to give a trial of treatment before calling in the "superspecialist." We think, with a few guidelines that most physicians did not learn in medical school, they can function the same way with the psychosocial problems of pediatric patients.

Psychiatrists may worry that, if every physician wholeheartedly adopts the biopsychosocial developmental approach in practice, psychiatrists will have nothing to do except be caretakers of the most treatment-refractory situations. Such an occurrence seems theoretically possible, and realistically improbable. Time and schedule always limit the number of children with emotional problems whom the pediatrician can accept as his patients. Of necessity, he or she must refer the others, and child psychiatrists need to inspire enough confidence to permit the pediatrician to make these referrals comfortably. As the pediatricians gain proficiency in helping these children, their referrals to the child psychiatrists will carry a higher percentage of very difficult or even treatment-refractory situations. However, it seems inevitable that, as child psychiatrists and pediatricians work more closely together, the child psychiatrist will benefit from an increasing number of interesting and very treatable children rather than fewer referrals.

SUMMARY

The interface between pediatrics and child psychiatry has not been ideal. In the last three decades, both professions have moved toward each other and have been actively seeking ways of working together for the most benefit to the most children in the community.

I do not subscribe to either extreme view that the pediatrician should treat all childhood behavior problems or that he/she should never treat such problems. I am very skeptical of the benefit society might obtain from the establishment of a new subspecialty in behavioral pediatrics. I prefer that all primary physicians become competent in biopsychosocial, developmental medicine. A seven-item "Prognosis Guide" is offered to assist in selecting cases best suited for office therapy by the primary care physician. In using this guide, both the pediatrician and the child psychiatrist should become able to work together on appropriately selected cases, identify those problems that can be effectively managed by the pediatrician and decide which children need total psychiatric care.

REFERENCES

1. Hamilton, N.G. and Sack, W.H.: An evaluation survey of a pediatric child psychiatry liaison program, paper read at the Annual Meeting of the American Academy of Child Psychiatry, Fall 1977.
2. Kempe, C.H. (Chairman): The future of pediatric education, a report by The Task Force on Pediatric Education, January 1976 through February 1978. Privately printed but unpublished.

3. Parcel, G.S., Nader, P.R., and Meyer, M.P.: Adolescent health concerns, problems and patterns of utilization in a triethnic urban population. Pediatr., *60*:157, 1977.
4. Rothenberg, M.B.: Child psychiatry-pediatrics liaison: A history and commentary. J. Am. Acad. Child Psychiatry, *7*:492, 1968.
5. Tarjan, G. et al. (Eds.): *The Physician and the Mental Health of the Child, III. Interrelating Primary Medical Practice and other Human Services.* Chicago, American Medical Association, 1981.

Index